Ethics and Midwifery

Issues in Contemporary Practice

SECOND EDITION

Lucy Frith BA(Hons) MPhil

Lecturer in Health Care Ethics, Department of Primary Care,
The University of Liverpool, UK

Heather Draper

Centre for Biomedical Ethics, Primary Care Building,
The Medical School, University of Birmingham, UK

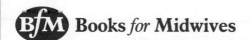 Books *for* Midwives

EDINBURGH LONDON NEW YORK OXFORD PHILADELPHIA ST LOUIS SYDNEY TORONTO 2004

BOOKS FOR MIDWIVES
An imprint of Elsevier Limited

First edition 1996
Second edition 2004
  Reprinted 2004

ISBN 0 7506 5350 7

British Library Cataloguing in Publication Data
A catalogue record for this book is available from the British Library

Library of Congress Cataloging in Publication Data
A catalog record for this book is available from the Library of Congress

Notice
Medical knowledge is constantly changing. Standard safety precautions must be followed, but as new research and clinical experience broaden our knowledge, changes in treatment and drug therapy may become necessary or appropriate. Readers are advised to check the most current product information provided by the manufacturer of each drug to be administered to verify the recommended dose, the method and duration of administration, and contraindications. It is the responsibility of the practitioner, relying on experience and knowledge of the patient, to determine dosages and the best treatment for each individual patient. Neither the Publisher nor the editor/contributor assumes any liability for any injury and/or damage to persons or property arising from this publication.

The Publisher

 ELSEVIER your source for books, journals and multimedia in the health sciences
www.elsevierhealth.com

The publisher's policy is to use paper manufactured from sustainable forests

Printed in China

Contents

List of contributors

Rebecca Bennett BA(Hons), PhD
*Lecturer in Bioethics, Centre for Social Ethics and Policy,
School of Law, University of Manchester, UK*

Martien Brands MD, PhD
*Senior Clinical Lecturer in Homeopathy, Department of
Primary Care, University of Liverpool, UK*

Rachel Clarke MA(Medical Ethics), RM, ADM, MTD/Cert Ed
*Was a lecturer in Midwifery Studies and is now a reflexologist and
healer, working in Norwich*

Soo Downe BA, RM, MSc, PhD
*Director, Midwifery Studies Research Unit, University of Central
Lancashire, UK*

Heather Draper BA(Hons), MA(Thesis), PhD
*Senior Lecturer in Biomedical Ethics, Centre for Biomedical Ethics,
University of Birmingham, UK*

Lucy Frith BA(Hons), MPhil
*Lecturer in Health Care Ethics, Department of Primary Care,
University of Liverpool, UK*

Carolyn Hicks BA, MA, PhD, PGCE, CPsychol
Professor of Health Psychology, University of Birmingham, UK

Janet Holt MPhil, BA(Hons), PGDip, RGN, RM, ADM, RTN
Lecturer, School of Health Studies, University of Leeds, UK

David Lamb BA, PhD
*Honorary Reader in Bioethics, Centre for Biomedical Ethics,
University of Birmingham, UK*

Alison Ledward BA, RGN, RM, MSc
*Research Student (MPhil), Department of Primary Care,
University of Liverpool, UK*

Rosemary Mander MSc, PhD, RGN, SCM, MTD
Reader, School of Nursing Studies, University of Edinburgh, UK

Hazel McHaffie PhD, SRN, RM
*Deputy Director of Research, Institute of Medical Ethics,
University of Edinburgh, UK*

Jean McHale LLb(Hons), MPhil
Professor of Law, Faculty of Law, University of Leicester, UK

Pam Miller SRN, SCM, MA, DN, Cert. Ed.
*Clinical Educator, Neonatal Unit, Birmingham Women's
Hospital, UK*

Catherine Williams SRN, HVCert, SCM, BA(Hons)
*Lecturer in Women's Health, Department of Primary Health Care,
University College of St. Martin, Lancaster, UK*

Introduction
Heather Draper

When the first edition of this collection was written, many of the contributors, and the editor in her introduction, anticipated that midwifery was about to be radically changed for the better by the introduction of different working practices recommended by *Changing Childbirth* (DoH 1993). The professional status of midwives was set to be enhanced because midwives would be considered the 'lead-professional—undertaking the key role in the planning and provision of care' (DoH 1993), particularly in the case of uncomplicated pregnancies and deliveries. Not surprisingly many midwives believed that *Changing Childbirth* would re-establish them as autonomous professionals in their own right, and redefine the professional boundaries between midwifery and obstetrics. *Changing Childbirth* also recognised the need for pregnant and labouring women to regain some of their autonomy too, by promising that women would have more choice in the way in which their pregnancy and labour were managed: an initiative called women-centred care. In addition, there was a commitment that maternity services 'should be readily and easily accessible to all. They should be sensitive to the needs of the local population and based primarily in the community' (DoH 1993). These twin changes—midwifery-led care and women-centred care—suggested that in the near future midwives and women would be able to forge new partnerships based on mutual respect and an acknowledgment that pregnancy and labour are, in the majority of cases, part of the normal pattern of health for women who choose to have babies. Frith (1996) noted that the recommendations implied 'a degree of ethical sophistication ... from practitioners ... [through] increased decision-making capacity ... and more ethical responsibility for the patient'.

A friend recently had her third child and her experience was far removed from the service promised in *Changing Childbirth*. Her first labour (in the UK) ended in a caesarean section. Her second pregnancy resulted in successful vaginal delivery (in Australia), but because of her history of caesarean section, and some problems with the second baby shortly after she was born, when my friend returned to the UK pregnant for a third time she was happy to agree to have this baby in a hospital. Unfortunately, during the time that she was out of the country, her local maternity ward had closed, and the service had been centralised to a larger hospital some distance away. When she went, at the invitation of the midwives, to visit this hospital delivery suite she was informed that there was no guarantee that a midwife would be with her during the whole of her labour as it was usual for midwives to be busy, often with two, sometimes three, labouring women at the same time. Other services, like water birthing, had been withdrawn. Reluctantly, my friend decided to hire a doula. This turned out to be a wise choice because labour progressed very quickly and most of it was spent in the car battling with rush-hour traffic to get to the hospital (to deliver in a safe environment!). Her husband was driving and becoming alarmed about the traffic, directions to the hospital, and the prospect of his wife delivering in the car, but the doula was able to keep my friend calm and focused. The baby was born within 5 minutes of getting to the hospital. For my friend, choice had to be purchased and services felt far from local.

Studies have shown that women-centred care, continuity of care and midwifery-led services—central to *Changing Childbirth*—are popular with women (Page et al 1999, Spurgeon et al 2001, Fleissig et al 1996). Yet according to Jowett (1998) and Taylor (2000), Trusts have generally avoided embracing change as either too expensive or lacking in evidence of effectiveness. Ten years on and many women and midwives are still waiting for the paradigm shift in maternity services to occur, and both may be disappointed by the slow speed of progress. Certainly, judging by some of the contributions in this collection, the much-heralded revolution in midwifery has failed to materialise in a way that has enhanced the professional status or autonomy of midwives (see for instance, Ledward, Chapter 13).

So why have a second edition? *Changing Childbirth* did imply revolutionised services and more professional autonomy for midwives, but even without these changes midwifery is a profession with its own responsibilities, ethical duties and ethical problems. Some aspects of midwifery have changed, even though these changes were not quite what was expected. Many midwives now have extended roles, though this is arguably as much a result of changing working practices for junior doctors as an attempt to provide midwife-led services. It could be argued that these extended roles have further blurred the boundaries between obstetrics and midwifery, or it could be argued that they have enhanced the status of midwives by giving them more responsibility. Also, the expectations of women have been raised, not just by *Changing Childbirth*, but also by the rise in consumerism in health care services generally. Moreover, midwifery was not a profession that lacked ethics or ethical problems prior to *Changing Childbirth*. Interest in ethical issues continues to rise, both in the general population (as evidenced by ethical consumerism and popular media programmes centring either on an ethical dilemma or the ethical integrity of the participants) and in the caring professions generally. Writing for specific professions and professional interests has become common, with books and journals dedicated to ethics in business, accountancy, law, insurance, nursing, individual special-ties of medicine (obstetrics, anaesthetics, paediatrics, etc), journal-ism, universities, policing and food production to name but a few. It is recognised that even though in some aspects ethics rightly comes in a 'one size fits all' form (the need to respect autonomy, avoid avoidable harm, honesty, confidentiality, etc.), practical ethics is most helpful when it can be very specific, address the special con-cerns of individuals and take account of their professional con-straints, working environment and issues that are commonly faced. Even without a revolution in the midwifery profession, there is still a need for a collection addressing the distinctive problems faced by midwives.

THE DISTINCTIVE CONCERNS OF MIDWIFERY

There are several distinctive concerns of midwifery: (i) there are at least two patients in the carer/patient relationship; (ii) at least one of these patients is usually going through a normal process that has no associations with illness or disease (and this is recognised in the phil-osophy of midwifery care); (iii) midwifery has a tradition of profes-sional autonomy which is often frustrated by the medicalisation (and therefore obstetricalisation) of pregnancy and childbirth; and (iv) (partly for this reason) midwives often have to be team players in a team where professional hierarchies are unclear or in dispute. These concerns are not unique to midwifery, but combined they cre-ate the working environment that generates many of the common ethical issues that face modern midwifery as a profession and in practice. As such, these defining features are themes throughout this collection.

i. Two (or more) in one

Midwives have equal responsibility for the woman and the foetus—the Midwives Code of Practice (UKCC 1998) states that '[t]he needs of the mother and baby must be the primary focus of your practice'. In the majority of cases this presents little if any conflict of interests as what is best for the mother is best for the fetus and vice versa. There are then some grey areas where small risks of minor harm are generally agreed to be outweighed by small benefits to one party or other, or even where certain small harms are outweighed by predicted benefits. A common example here would be that women tolerate unpleasant morning sickness and nausea because the drugs that would remove this unpleasantness may cause harm to the fetus. Mander, in Chapter 3, discusses a more complex version of this kind of case, the use of mobile epidurals. Mobile epidurals are more likely to result in a vaginal delivery than the traditional epidural, but they are also associated with poorer neonatal condition at birth. More difficult are cases where real and immediate harm to one party or the other has to be balanced against more significant benefits—as in the case of an emergency caesarean prompted by fetal distress (see Draper, Chapter 1 and McHale, Chapter 2). Equally difficult are cases where the understanding of benefit is open to dispute, for instance late termination in the case of fetal impairment (see Holt, Chapter 8).

It is rarely the case that a midwife practising in developed countries is charged with the responsibility of choosing between the life of the woman or the life of the fetus. Chris Bohjalian's fictional and ambiguous account of one such situation in *Midwives* (1998) gives a graphic insight into the tensions caused both by such a decision; and by one made by a midwife in a profession jealously dominated by obstetricians. Traditionally, midwives have given greatest weight to the life of the woman. This is partly because the fetus, even at the point of birth, does not have the same legal (and arguably moral—see Lamb, Chapter 9) status as the woman (see McHale, Chapter 2), and partly for the pragmatic historical reasons that women often had existing children whose needs were also taken into account, because babies born to dead mothers were unlikely to survive, and because if the woman survived she could hope to have another child in the future. Nevertheless, in practice midwifery tends to err on the side of preserving fetal life and health at the cost of the health of the mother, and most women on most occasions would be happy to accept this balance. But it remains a balance, and it is one that means that midwives (in common with obstetricians and obstetric anaesthetists) do have potentially directly conflicting duties to patients who are inextricably linked.

ii. Pregnancy and birth as a normal process

The philosophy of midwifery has always encompassed the view that pregnancy and birth are normal, and the care given should not therefore be modelled on that which is appropriate in the case of illness or disease. Midwives are the experts in this normal process, and arguably their primary role is to act as experienced and skilled companions to women at this time (Page 1995). Midwives are also trained to recognise cases that deviate from the norm enough to warrant obstetric advice. The emphasis is important: midwives start from the position that pregnancy and labour are normal, and not from the position that they are normal in retrospect (for a fuller discussion of this theme, see Downe, Chapter 5). For this reason, midwives have both different care strategies and different ends to other health care practitioners. The midwife's care strategy can be one of facilitating genuine choice (as the woman is not ill and in this respect her autonomy is not compromised by ill health) and making the experience as pleasant as possible. A woman's experience of birth can affect the way she feels about and adapts to motherhood, so it is important that this is as rewarding an experience as possible. Birth is not an unpleasant means to an end in the same way an operation is. An operation is a necessary evil and pain is minimised to reduce this evil as much as possible. In labour pain is part of the normal process and can be useful, albeit unpleasant. Midwives are trained both to accept pain and to help labouring women cope with it, but also to recognise when pain has become unproductive. Pain itself has a different meaning than in other health care contexts, it is part of the process and not purely an undesirable side effect or symptom (see, for instance, Brands, Chapter 11). Midwives also have different ends for their practice, their goal is not to cure but to help facilitate a natural event and to prepare the woman for parenthood and a radical future change in lifestyle.

iii. Frustration of professional autonomy

Having a profession is often associated with having a professional body that acts as gatekeeper for entry to the profession in terms of training, examination, ongoing registration and professional standards (which disciplinary measures—including being excluded from the profession—maintain). In this sense, the profession itself defines and polices its own professional boundaries: in essence it defines itself and seeks public recognition and respect for what it has defined as its own. Professional autonomy is thereby limited, by necessity, to the profession that one professes to be a part of and should not be confused with autonomy per se. Midwives cannot claim to have *professional* autonomy to eat whatever they choose, but as autonomous individuals they can certainly make such decisions for themselves. Professional autonomy refers to the freedom to exercise judgement related to one's profession within the bounds of one's professional expertise. A midwife cannot claim to be entitled as a matter of professional autonomy to decide whether to perform a caesarean section or to let a more junior member of staff perform it. The performing of caesarean sections does not fall within the professional boundaries of midwifery, neither does brick laying or electrical installation or the representation of one's client in a court. Thus professional autonomy is not constrained when one is not permitted to do any of these things as a midwife, and nor does professional autonomy extend to acting in a way that is considered to be negligent by the profession.

The frustration of professional autonomy occurs when a professional is not permitted to exercise appropriate professional judgement while working as that professional. One of the difficulties facing midwifery is how the boundaries of the profession are defined and who should define them (see Clarke, Chapter 12). This is not just a problem for midwifery, it is true of nursing and to some extent anaesthetics too. As a profession, midwifery ought to define its own boundaries and professional responsibilities but this is often something that has to be negotiated with other professions who also have a professional interest (for instance, obstetrics and paediatrics) and as a result, some of the professional boundaries have become blurred. This means that at these boundaries, professional autonomy is also unclear.

Medicine as a profession is very hierarchical, and so too is health care delivery with doctors generally located at the top of the pecking order. In turn, this means that obstetricians sometimes feel that they have the professional autonomy to *override* the professional judgement of a midwife; indeed, they may feel that they have a duty to override what they perceive as an incorrect judgement. They may also believe that it is best to have systems in place that ensure that they, rather than the midwives, have the final say where the boundaries of professional responsibility are blurred. This is understandable and even justifiable where their legal responsibilities are greater. However, because of the existence of the overall hierarchy, it is possible for this process to be much more casual than it needs to be, and than one would otherwise expect it to be when the judgement of two *professionals* is at issue. For instance, two consultants from different specialties would automatically expect that where there was a differ-ence of professional judgement about a patient in their dual care this would be open for courteous professional discussion that led to shared agreement, not one consultant overriding or disregarding the views of another. This would be expected not just as a matter of pro-fessional etiquette but also as a matter of ethical responsibility when the best interests of the patient are at stake, and uncertain to the extent that there is room for professional disagreement.

Similarly, where a midwife's professional judgement is over-ridden in a way that is casual and disrespectful there is cause for legitimate complaint where there are systems in place that limit legitimate professional judgement (see Ledward, Chapter 13). There is less cause for complaint when legal responsibility is not equally shared, unless the midwife has the greater responsibility. Similarly, midwives must be cautious to distinguish between professional autonomy and the autonomy that they have as persons. An example here is the exercise of the conscience clauses that are found in both the Abortion Act 1967 and the Human Fertilisation and Embryology Act 1992. When a midwife refuses to perform some procedure on the grounds of conscience, this is not as a result of professional judgement, but rather an expression of personal autonomy. At other times, personal autonomy does not have such a free rein in the context of professional obligations.

Anyone asserting what they see to be their rights using the con-cept of autonomy must be mindful of the fact that autonomy is a double-edged sword. To be autonomous is certainly to be able to exercise choice, but it is also to be held responsible—accountable—for the choices that have been made. It is unfair to be held accountable for situations over which one has no control, and it is also for this reason that it would be unfair for one professional to insist on mak-ing a decision, and then to expect or allow another professional to take responsibility if things go wrong as a result.

iv. Working in a team

This leads directly on from the discussion of professional autonomy in that team working requires both cooperation and respect for each member's expertise.

> The highest priority should be given to the care of women and infants. This means that all members of the maternity care team should recognise and value their own and each other's particular

skills and contribution, but equally be prepared to work flexibly in order to ensure that the needs of families are met. (Royal College of Midwives 2002)

It is not only midwives who complain about attempts, successful or otherwise, to frustrate their professional autonomy. Scott (2003) writes about the interprofessional conflicts that can arise between midwives and anaesthetists about the siting of an epidural, for while it is the midwives who use their judgement to request that an epidural is sited, the anaesthetists are responsible for it during the time that it is in place and for any complications that arise afterwards. Accordingly, anaesthetists have to decide whether an epidural can be safely used, given the condition of the woman, the staffing situation and other commitments at the time, and this may mean refusing to accede to the request on the grounds that it is not safe to do so. In Scott's view, anaesthetists are sometimes treated as though they are technicians rather than professionals in their own right, too.

On one reading of Scott, her point is not that the anaesthetist overrides the professional autonomy of the midwife, but rather that the midwife's professional autonomy only extends to requesting that an epidural be sited, based on judging how labour is progressing and what the woman herself wants and needs. It can both be the case that the midwife was right to request the epidural and that one could not be safely sited, in the equally right judgement of the anaesthetist, because there were insufficient staff to ensure that it could be monitored properly. Each person has to respect the professionalism of the other.

But teams are not always composed of professional equals. Midwifery teams, for instance, may contain nursing assistants, trainees, recently qualified midwives, midwives new to the specialty and very experienced and senior midwives. Other teams may comprise midwives, obstetricians, anaesthetists and paediatricians of differing levels of seniority and experience. The difficulty of team working is highlighted when controversial decisions have to be made and implemented (see Miller, Chapter 7). Allowing 'one member one vote' does not solve the ethical problems, as situations could easily arise where just under half of the members of the team are implementing a decision with which they are in professional disagreement. Awarding only one person decision-making responsibilities may also mean that some people are implementing a decision with which they disagree, and they may also feel that they had no say in this decision—which cannot be said in the case of 'one person one vote'. On the other hand, if it is the most senior person who carries the burden of legal responsibilities, is it right that this individual's neck is put on the line for a decision with which he or she did not agree but which the rest of the team wanted? Consensus team decision-making can lead to half-measures being taken, because they are less controversial, and these might also not be in the interests of the patient. Nor is it obvious that teams work best when only the senior members participate in decision-making, the outcomes of which have to be implemented by the whole team. At the very least, all members of the team should have had the opportunity to be heard (not just to speak) and should understand the rationale behind the decision, even if it remains one with which they cannot agree.

Last but not least, one would normally expect that a competent patient was a full member of the team.

This brief introduction to the distinctive concerns of midwifery also indicates where some of the chapters in this collection deal in more detail with these concerns. Other chapters also fit within these themes, but more loosely. Obviously some chapters deal with one or possibly two of these themes in detail, none addresses all of them, but it is worthwhile bearing them all in mind when reading through the collection.

OUTLINE OF THE CONTENTS

The collection gives a broad overview of the many ethical problems that midwives could face in practice. It is not intended to be an introduction to moral theory, rather it raises issues in their practical context to demonstrate the tensions and conflicts that exist, enabling realistic solutions and approaches to be formulated. Many of the authors are practising midwives, the rest are academic specialists in health care ethics, medical law, health psychology and homeopathy. Only two of the chapters in the collection appear much as they did in the 1996 edition (McHaffie, Chapter 15 and Williams, Chapter 6). One has been updated by the editors (Clarke, Chapter 12). The remainder have either been substantially updated or completely rewritten by the authors, or are new chapters specially commissioned to complement the collection. Lucy Frith was responsible for conceiving the book and for all the commissioning. Heather Draper was responsible for the editing.

The volume is divided into three sections; Everyday issues, Technological issues and Professional issues, with cross-referencing throughout the chapters so that links can be made. Inevitably some subjects will not be covered and some views not expressed. Some chapters take the form of providing a general introduction to a subject, and in others the author develops a line of thought that represents his or her personal view. One volume cannot possibly cover all the ethical issues midwives might face, but ways of approaching problems are indicated and these can be applied to those issues not raised.

The first section, Everyday issues, examines some of the ethical problems that are central and common in midwifery practice. These issues are mundane in the sense that they are everyday, but can be no less acute and disturbing when they arise in practice. Heather Draper considers the general issue of consent in childbirth in Chapter 1, with a broad introduction to the issue of consent that discusses the theoretical basis of the concept and its four elements of competence, information, voluntariness and decision. She then goes on to consider the practical importance of consent and examines the possible conflicts that could arise if the woman pursues a course of action that is likely to bring harm to herself or if she refuses consent for treatment that might be in the best interests of the fetus (introducing the 'two (or more) patients in one' theme). This chapter provides a theoretical backdrop to subsequent discussions on consent.

In Chapter 2, Jean McHale provides an introduction to the midwife's legal obligations during pregnancy, the birth and postnatally. Also picking up the theme that both fetus and woman have interests, she outlines the legal status of the fetus and asks what restraints on the pregnant woman in the interests of the fetus might be legal, particularly since the introduction of the Human Rights Act 1998. During her section on the birth, she describes the midwife's duty of care and discusses the case law related to performing caesarean sections without consent in the interests of the fetus. In the final section, she warns that once the fetus is born alive, he or she becomes a patient in his or her own right, and midwives may then, in various circumstances that she outlines, have a duty to act in the interests of the child against the wishes of the parents.

Chapter 3 extends the discussion about consent to specific clinical interventions in labour, focusing primarily on epidural analgesia in uncomplicated labour. Rosemary Mander considers the likelihood of two salient features of consent (information and voluntariness) being feasible in the context of epidural analgesia and other interventions in labour such as caesarean section and episiotomy. She suggests that intervention rates might be due more to the practices of individual midwifes than the needs of particular women and the choices they make. She concludes that the acceptance of epidural services has been fostered by the expectation that mothers will fail to cope with the pain of uncomplicated labour and that further research is needed into pain control and ways of increasing women's expectation of coping with pain so that such a service can be provided on an ethical basis.

Routine antenatal testing for HIV is discussed by Rebecca Bennett in Chapter 4. Bennett is concerned with how to balance the need to respect the autonomy and choices of pregnant women against testing for HIV as a public health measure, where success is measured in terms of uptake (the higher the better on the grounds of utility, where the interests of the individual have to be balanced against the protection of others from avoidable harm). She notes that if pressure to accept testing is justified in terms of prevention and cure, then if a woman tests positive, she is likely to come under further pressure to accept treatment. Bennett analyses the evidence that is used to reinforce the ethical principle of utility and finds that it is not as compelling as it seems at first glance. She is also concerned that if coercive measures are justified in the case of HIV infection, similar arguments could be used to justify other restrictions on the choices of pregnant women for the benefit of the fetus. She concludes that the debate over routine antenatal testing for HIV needs to become more transparent so that proper choices can be made about how to balance the ethical principles at stake. Her conclusions are readily transferable to other areas of routine screening.

Chapters 5 and 6 broaden the discussion to cover general underlying themes of relevance to all pregnancy and childbirth. These chapters address philosophical aspects of childbirth, i.e. how we theorise about it, how it is conceptualised and elaborating on the ethical and practical dimensions of adopting these theoretical positions. In Chapter 5 Soo Downe examines the concept of normality. Midwives are trained to be experts in normal childbirth and any deviation from the norm must be referred to a medical practitioner. Given that once a woman is referred to an obstetrician, her pregnancy and delivery are likely to become more medicalised, it becomes important to have a clear idea about what is meant by normality—both for the sake of the woman concerned and for the sake of maintaining the integrity of the midwifery profession. This is a debate in which midwives should take the lead and formulate a definition of normality based on good research and practical evidence. Downe considers definitions of abnormality and risk, the effects such definitions have on pregnant women and the professional implications for midwives. In so doing she opens discussion on the themes that pregnancy is normal and how the midwifery profession can maintain its professional autonomy and work with related practitioners.

In Chapter 6 Catherine Williams' consideration of the relationship between sexuality, the reproductive continuum and the midwife continues these themes. The increasing medicalisation of childbirth has separated sexuality from the birth process and reduced midwives to coy maiden birth attendants. Williams argues that if sexuality is excluded from the birth process, rather than making it safer, it actually complicates and confuses the relationship between the midwife and mother. By conceptualising birth as a medical event, the diversity of women's needs is not recognised, forcing women to experience birth in a predetermined way. She claims that midwives need to recognise and acknowledge the sexual nature of childbirth in order to be able to relate honestly to, and support, the person seeking professional assistance.

The second section, Technological issues, examines some of the ethical dilemmas created by technological interventions in pregnancy and reproduction more generally. Some of the issues raised in this section will have a direct bearing on midwifery practice; others will be of more general interest so that midwives can be kept informed of wider ethical issues.

Chapter 7 considers the ethical issues raised in neonatal intensive care. Pam Miller examines the ethical problems that can arise, such as whether every live-born baby should be offered full intensive care and how this decision should be reached, the criteria to be used for withdrawing care and whether and how babies with genetic disorders should be treated. Finally, the problem of resources and staffing is addressed and Miller concludes that practitioners must each develop their own ethical stance on the issues raised so that they can provide the best possible care for their patients. Her use of case studies also illustrates that the patient (or in the case of children, the parent(s)) is part of the team who have to make decisions they can all live with, and the theme of team working is a recurrent one in this chapter.

Chapter 8 takes up points briefly considered by Miller and Downe as it focuses on the question of what should happen when an impairment is detected by an ultrasound scan. Janet Holt considers the wider issues raised by screening, such as whether people should be allowed to choose the kind of baby they have and the implications of genetic screening for the individual and society. She widens this discussion still further to include screening at the preimplantation stage. She is interested in the relationships between screening and eugenics and is concerned that slippery slopes should be avoided.

In Chapter 9 David Lamb first considers the leading arguments for and against the use of fetal tissue transplantation, building on the discussion of abortion developed in Holt's chapter. The separation principle is examined, which claims that the alleged benefits of fetal transplantation can be separated from what some people see as the stigma of voluntary abortion. The chapter looks at the issue of who should consent for the transplants, examines how the fetus is conceptualised and suggests how fetal tissue could be used in an ethically acceptable way. Lamb next discusses the related issue of stem cell research, which is currently legal in the UK but which the European Parliament (at the time of writing) is considering banning completely. He considers in some detail the moral standing of the human embryo and suggests that the use of the '3 Rs' (a notion borrowed from animal research) might help to govern research on human embryos given that their moral standing remains a matter of dispute. This chapter provides much in the way of theoretical background to issues in research, the status of the embryo/fetus, and the use of human tissue in research.

In Chapter 10 Lucy Frith introduces some of the recurrent ethical issues that arise in the use of reproductive technologies, such as who should be given access to these technologies, the status of the embryo, cloning and what the children born as a result of these treatments should be told. She considers the legislative provisions and the role of the Human Fertilisation and Embryology Authority (HFEA). The chapter concludes with an indication of practical ethical difficulties that pregnancies conceived in this way can create for the midwife involved in their management.

In the introduction, the point was made that professionals have to determine their own boundaries, and where these boundaries fall has an impact on those working in related areas. In Chapter 11, Martien Brands aims to convince us that the use of homeopathy is compatible with the practice of midwifery, and the philosophy and goals of the midwifery profession. He gives examples of how homeopathy could be safely introduced and how it has been incorporated in the Netherlands. He suggests that it may also promote the autonomy of women, as it may be used to facilitate more low intervention home births. Homeopathy is not generally a technique that one associates with 'technology', but rather with alternative and complementary therapies, but this chapter does not sit uneasily in this section as a 'new' intervention.

The final section, Professional issues, concentrates on the possible constraints on midwives' professional autonomy and considers the codes of practice and the professional obligations that delineate midwifery practice. The section also examines the ethics of research, as midwives have a professional obligation to ensure that their practice is evidence-based, which in its turn means that it is increasingly common for midwives to be involved in research.

Chapter 12 provides a critical view of the code of practice that governs nursing and midwifery. Rachel Clarke argues that the code of professional conduct is unjust in its expectations as it assumes that midwives are autonomous practitioners when in practice they are unable to exercise such autonomy. Clarke contends that the contrast between the myth of professional freedom and the observed control of midwives by employers, medicine and the state exposes the fallibility of the midwives' belief about their status in 20th-century childbearing. She claims that the code, in assuming such professional autonomy, thus encourages midwives to make autonomous judgements but punishes them if they do in fact act autonomously.

In Chapter 13 Alison Ledward continues the theme of professional autonomy. She argues that the changes promised in *Changing Midwifery* suggested greater professional autonomy for midwifery but that this has failed to materialise. Instead, professional autonomy has been frustrated, leading to a retention crisis in midwifery. She gives many examples of the ways in which this process has occurred, and points out that some of the measures thought to increase professional autonomy might even be counter to the philosophy of midwifery because they promote technical skills that are associated with the medicalisation of childbearing. Her chapter inevitably also includes the theme of interprofessional working.

The final two chapters focus on the issue of research. Chapter 14 gives a broad introduction to the ethical problems raised by conducting a research project and offers practical advice on elements that should be considered when formulating an ethical research proposal. Concentrating specifically on research in midwifery, Carolyn Hicks considers the ethical aspects of questions such as: What is the research topic? Who is to conduct the research? Who will benefit from the research? Where will the research be conducted? How will the participants be treated? How will the research be carried out? How will the findings be disseminated? She includes an ethical appraisal of the use of the randomised control trial as the 'gold standard' for current research practice. Chapter 15 develops in more detail some of the issues addressed by Hicks and considers the possible ethical problems raised by researching sensitive information. Hazel McHaffie introduces the problems, such as maintaining confidentiality and handling distressing information, by citing examples taken from her own research experience. The chapter gives practitioners an idea of the constraints on researchers as well as alerting would-be researchers to some of the possible pitfalls.

Although the collection cannot give definitive answers to the ethical dilemmas and tensions encountered in practice, by raising issues and engaging in discussion, progress towards consensus and resolution can be hastened. Open discussion of ethical issues can reduce the sense of isolation many practitioners feel when confronted with ethical problems. It is useful to discuss thought processes and reasons for acting so that these can be opened up to scrutiny, enabling the elimination of bad practice and the promotion and applauding of good practice.

References

Bohjalian C 1998 Midwives. Vintage, London

Department of Health 1993 Changing childbirth. HMSO, London

Fleissig A, Kroll D, McCarthy M 1996 Is community-led midwifery care a feasible option for women assessed at low risk and those with complicated pregnancies? Results for a population study based in South Camden, London. Midwifery 12:191–197

Frith L 1996 Introduction. In Frith L (ed) Ethics and midwifery. Butterworth-Heinemann, Oxford

Jowett M 1998 Small change. Midwifery Matters 77. Online. Available: www.radmid.demon.co.uk

Page L et al 1999 Clinical interventions and outcomes of one-to-one midwifery practice. Journal of Public Health Medicine 21:243–248

Page L 1995 Putting principles into practice. In Page L (ed) Effective group practice in midwifery. Blackwell, Oxford

Royal College of Midwives 2002 Position paper 26 Refocusing the role of the midwife. Online. Available: www.rcm.org.uk

Scott W 2003 Maternal foetal conflicts and the anaesthetist's role. In Draper H, Scott W (eds) Ethics in anaesthesia and intensive care. Elsevier, Oxford

Spurgeon P, Hicks C, Barwell F 2001 Antenatal, delivery and postnatal comparisons of maternal satisfaction with two pilot Changing Childbirth schemes, compared with a traditional model of care. Midwifery 17:123–132

Taylor M 2000 Is midwifery dying? Midwifery Matters 84. Online. Available: www.radmid.demon.co.uk

United Kingdom Central Council (UKCC) 1998 Midwives rules and code of practice. Online. Available: www.nmc-uk.org

PART 1

Everyday issues

PART CONTENTS

Chapter 1

Ethics and consent in midwifery

Heather Draper

INTRODUCTION

This chapter will look at how the process of gaining consent is justi-fied in ethical theory. It will then examine some of the circumstances in which gaining or respecting consent can cause ethical problems for midwives.

CONSENT AND AUTONOMY

Respect for autonomy can be found in two contrasting ideas from moral theory. The first is that autonomy is inextricably linked to responsibility and flows from the control we are able to exercise over our will. There are some things over which we cannot exercise our will. We cannot for instance choose to fall in love. In that sense we are not responsible for who we love or other feelings we may have, but we are of course responsible for how we choose to act on those feelings. If a person chooses to do one thing rather than another then that person can, and should, be held responsible for the decision. If, however, the person was forced to do one thing when he or she would have chosen to do another, then it would be unfair to hold that person responsible for the action over which he or she had no control. He or she did not make the decision; the person applying the force made it. It is the willing choice of one course of action when another could have been followed that gives us responsibility: where autonomous choice is exercised, responsibility follows. Without the capacity to will our own behaviour we could have no notion of moral responsibility (like animals, we would only act instinctively) and in this sense, autonomy is valuable for without it there could be no ethics. To respect an individual's autonomy is therefore to respect their moral agency.

The second reason to respect autonomy is based on the contention that without individual autonomy there can be no individual innovation and without individual innovation society would stagnate. Innovators often challenge the status quo in a way that members of it find disturbing, but we need to be tolerant of an individual's liberty not to conform because non-conformists can change attitudes, behaviours, science and technology in a way that is ultimately beneficial for everyone. An individual's liberty should, however, be constrained by the liberty and autonomy of others. This justification for respecting autonomy rests on the assumption that living in society is a good thing and that to remain good, societies must adapt and change.

Consent is closely associated with autonomy. To act on someone's body without their consent would be to undermine their autonomy, so gaining consent before doing anything to someone is a manifestation of respect for their autonomy and giving consent to a health care intervention is a legitimate expression of autonomy. When, however, patients consent to a procedure, while this is an expression of their responsibility for themselves as autonomous agents, it also follows that each patient must take responsibility for the course of action chosen. Part of taking responsibility is that one cannot blame others for the consequences flowing from the choice: to be responsible for making a choice means that one both makes the choice and is then accountable for the choice made.

Consent is also a safeguard for the patient's best interests. It is not unreasonable to assume that, given the choice, individuals will only choose to do that which is best for them. Moreover, individuals are in the best position to define for themselves that which is best for them. However, as Gillon (1986) points out, justifying respect for consent with reference to promotion of patients' best interests can have the effect of undermining patient autonomy. If serving their best interests is the end for which consent is the means and patients insist on a course of action that is not in their best interests, there is no longer a reason to respect their consent (or refusal of consent), and the end of serving their best interests would be better served by not allowing them to decide. The obvious response to this potential outcome is that there is no one objective measure of best interests and for this reason what is 'best' can be determined only by the individuals concerned: they alone are the judge of what is best for them. Acting to prevent what they want would be to impose one's own values and beliefs and these may not be right for the patient concerned; the paternalistic action would, therefore, be self-defeating. This is, however, a conclusion that is easier to agree in theory than in practice. What the midwife does or does not do in a situation such as this one contributes to the overall outcome, for instance, respecting the patient's wishes and not giving a life-saving blood transfusion or not performing an episiotomy to prevent a tear through to the anus. Even if one accepts the theoretical justification for respecting patient autonomy, the practical delivery of respect can be emotionally very tough.

To evaluate the imperative to respecting consent, we have to think about the relative value of autonomy. Does respect for autonomy, and therefore consent, have absolute value (i.e. it should never be overridden no matter what is in the balance) or is it very important but only relatively valuable (i.e. there are some circumstances where autonomy seems less important compared with other things to be weighed in the balance)? Absolute respect commits one to respect autonomy whatever the consequences might be. Relative respect allows for the possibility that on occasions it may be justifiable to override autonomy, but leaves one with the problems of determining what kinds of things are more important than autonomy and devising a system to apply the scale of value consistently.

Respect for autonomy does not mean that one must always do what someone wants simply because this is what they want. The ethical value of consent lies in giving patients the opportunity to refuse consent to something that they do not want. That a patient is willing to consent to a procedure does not mean that practitioners are obliged to carry out that procedure.

CONSENT AND PREGNANT WOMEN

In the case of pregnant women considerations about the value of consent are complicated by the presence within the woman of one or more fetuses. The discussion so far has assumed that there is one patient making a decision for herself, her body and her life. For a pregnant woman the health and life of the fetus may be directly affected by any decisions that she makes, particularly those related to her health. The extent to which the effects on the fetus matter morally will be influenced by views about its moral status, and whether it is likely to be born alive.

Some people believe that the fetus has no moral status and no interests until it is born. According to this view, there is no additional moral dimension to a pregnant woman's consent or refusal of consent, unless the fetus is born live but damaged as a result. If the fetus will go on to become a being that has interests in the future, and if these future interests will be damaged, arguably these interests have to be borne in mind. From this point of view, a decision that results in the death of a fetus matters less than one that results in it being born but harmed in some way. Nonetheless, even if the fetus is awarded interests, this does not mean that its interests count for more than anyone else's interests, principally the pregnant woman, but also perhaps her existing children, family and other commitments. But not everyone agrees about this; some women believe that it is right to put the interests of the fetus first, particularly if its life is at stake. This decision might be justified either by the belief that the fetus's right to life is equal to any other human, or because mothers have a special duty to protect the lives of their children. Different pregnant women will hold different views about the relative value of the fetus they are carrying, but acknowledging this may be of little practical help to midwives. Not only might individual practitioners have views about the status of the fetus that are different from their pregnant patients' views, but they may also feel professionally torn by having duties to both the women and the fetuses as *patients*, as midwifery has traditionally considered that both the woman and the fetus are legitimate subjects of their professional care.

All health care practitioners, whatever their background, have a professional obligation to serve the best interests of their patients, and as the fetus is also considered to be a patient, then in midwifery (as in other areas of practice) it is possible for there to be a direct conflict of interests between patients, and therefore a conflict of duties to patients. While all practitioners have to respect the autonomy of their pregnant patients, concerns have been raised about how this autonomy can and should be affected by the existence of the unborn fetus. The fetus is clearly not autonomous and is unable to express a point of view. Some midwives believe that while they have a duty to respect the autonomy of the pregnant patient, they must also safeguard the interests of the vulnerable fetus. This conflict will be explored in greater detail in the section of this chapter on the limits to autonomy.

WHAT CONSTITUTES CONSENT?

Legal precedent, a greater concern for ethical practice, greater awareness of the skill mixes in interrelated professions and Department of Health guidance, have all influenced the understanding of what it means to gain consent and give consent in the context of health service delivery. All practitioners and the majority of patients are now aware that consent is not a mere formality. In this chapter I have used the term 'consent' rather than 'informed consent' because the latter emphasises information but information is not the only element of consent, and if *any* element of consent is missing then consent has not been given or received. For an agreement to go on to constitute consent, the following four elements must have been satisfied: voluntariness, information, competence and decision.

Voluntariness

If an act is voluntary it is one that one has chosen for oneself without coercion. Clearly, though, the extent to which an action is voluntary also depends on how much information was received, whether or not one was deceived and also on one's ability to decide for oneself: voluntariness is therefore clearly related to the elements of competence and information. Freedom from coercion remains, however, an important element in its own right because of the difference in power between patients and professionals.

Coercion tends to be associated with threats of physical harm, like having a gun held to one's head, or the head of one's child. Such examples seem to have no parallel in health care. Whoever heard of patients being forced to have operations at gunpoint? It is, however, a mistake to think of coercion only in these terms. Coercion can be unsubtle without being violent and can be so subtle that it is hardly recognised as such.

An example of fairly unsubtle coercion is when a desired intervention is offered on condition that an undesired intervention is also accepted: for example, a termination of pregnancy will only be given if the woman also agrees to a concurrent sterilisation. Another fairly unsubtle way of coercing patients is the threat of withdrawing a desired intervention unless agreement to a further intervention is given. It is not, however, always the case that where one therapy is made dependent on another that coercion has occurred, but the line is a fine one. It may be that it is dangerous in a particular case to proceed with a surgical intervention unless the patient is also willing to agree to have a blood transfusion or an anaesthetic. It is not unreasonable for practitioners to exercise their own clinical judgement about how dangerous, or even effective, one intervention will be without another. But it would be unethical if the judgement being exercised is not clinical but one based on personal preference, prejudice, or ignorance. The difficulty lies in determining when the line from clinical judgement is crossed.

Practitioners ought not to be forced to compromise or prostitute their skills and judgement to whim—but how is whim to be determined in this context? For instance, when a woman requests a home delivery, her midwife also has to make a decision as a professional about how safe this is given the woman's circumstances, and how safe it is in the practitioner's hands. Some midwives would feel very uncomfortable about agreeing to deliver a baby at home because of their own lack of experience. In other cases, they may strongly believe that it is in the interests of the woman, and in the interests of a safe outcome for the baby, for the woman to have a hospital delivery. In the former case, no professional tension is caused by the midwife helping the woman to seek a midwife who does have the confidence and experience to manage a home birth. If, however, the midwife truly believes a home birth would be dangerous, that practitioner may also think that it is irresponsible to help the woman to take this risk by finding her another midwife. It is not unreasonable to refer a woman for a second opinion, but what if the midwife concerned *is* the second, third or even fourth opinion? Arguably, the refusal to get involved on the grounds of the risk to the woman is a form of coercion, since the most likely outcome if she cannot find a midwife is that she will be 'forced' to have a hospital delivery. This argument, however, requires an assessment of the extent to which running out of options constitutes coercion. The pregnant woman in this case may be being 'forced' by the consensus professional view of midwives to choose the hospital delivery, but it is not clear that if she has a hospital delivery she does so without her consent. This is not just because she could have 'chosen' to stay at home regardless (though realistically, this choice may now be closed to her) but rather that she does not have as many options as she thought she had. Her choices have been limited but she can still make some choices. The circumstances in which her choices have been limited, however, are also important for she would justifiably feel coerced if the midwives concerned were simply ignorant about the relative safety of home births, or just took a dislike to her. Respecting someone's autonomy does not, however, mean that they have to have everything they want, but rather that unreasonable constraints are not placed on what they are able to choose. Patients can also be coercive. A woman can, for instance, force a midwife to attend a home delivery whatever the risks, because she knows that midwives have a professional and legal obligation to provide emergency care even if this is in the home and against midwifery advice (Royal College of Midwives 2002).

Many women will be readily swayed by a midwife's opinion about what is best to do because their main preoccupation is to secure the best outcome for their babies. But being perceived as 'the expert' brings with it the responsibility only to pass considered judgements because comments made in passing may be given more weight than the midwife intended. This said, all practitioners should be free to express clinical judgement. It is not wrong for practitioners to tell patients that, in their opinion, a desired course of action is dangerous and to explain why this is so. As the Royal College of Midwives points out 'while it is important not to be perceived as bullying or coercive, it is important that women are not "protected" from understanding the possible implications of their decisions' (RCM 2002 p 3). It would, however, be coercive to withdraw all support unless and until some compromise agreement was reached. But while it is obvious to favour negotiation (for instance, to ask the woman what it is about a home delivery that cannot be provided by a hospital delivery and to try to accommodate these aspects within the hospital setting) there will from time to time be patients who, for one reason or another, will not meet in the middle ground (and undoubtedly, there are professionals like this too!). While these cases may prove the most memorable, it should not be forgotten that patients who are compliant are actually much more easily and routinely coerced than those who have strong views about what they want

Subtle coercion occurs more indirectly, often through verbal and nonverbal signals to the patient. Examples include treating a 'noncompliant' patient more brusquely than other patients, emphasising one therapy enthusiastically while mentioning genuine alternatives

y in passing, and confusing the patient with jargon or overloading
her with information. In midwifery, perhaps the most effective form
of subtle coercion is the suggestion, in the face of a patient's reluctance to agree, that harm might come to the baby if advice is ignored.
Tone of voice, tuts and hums can all be used to good effect to undermine a patient's confidence in her decision. Even here, though, there
is a difference between coercion and expressing an opinion as such,
or indeed making a recommendation in an environment where it is
possible for this recommendation to be rejected. The duty to inform
readily accommodates the expression of clinical judgement provided
that, where appropriate, practitioners make clear the extent to which
the verdict is an expression of their individual professional opinion
rather than the consensus view of their profession.

Information

Being informed is one aspect of acting in a way that is voluntary. This
mutual dependence is most vividly exemplified when a patient is
intentionally deceived. If a patient acts in ignorance of the truth, then
it is difficult to see how this decision can be described as voluntary,
particularly if, in the light of the information withheld, a different
decision would have been made. This is pretty clear-cut. Less obvious
is the amount of information that a patient requires in order to make
a decision. Too much information can paralyse a patient into indeci-
sion and anxiety, but then again this is an excuse readily offered by
those who prefer to make decisions for their patients. Determining
the amount of information a patient needs to make a decision is a
matter of professional judgement and balance made in good faith.
The minimum would be to discuss (in a language in which the
patient is fluent) options, risks and side-effects in the context of some
diagnosis and prognosis, in a jargon-free style, offering an opportunity for questions and including an assessment of the level of the
patient's understanding. But it is unrealistic to suggest that the
patient should be informed of every possible alternative therapy and
each and every conceivable side-effect or risk. What a patient requires
is enough relevant information to make a considered judgement.

Relevant information is that which facilitates autonomy—nothing
should be deliberately excluded that would influence the patient's
decision. Deliberately excluding information suggests an intention to
undermine autonomy through deception. It also suggests that the
midwife has a good understanding of what the woman needs to
know and because of this knowledge about the patient the midwife is

able to manipulate the situation. This is obviously unethical but it is also an enviable position for a midwife to be in. It would be much easier for midwives to discuss information honestly if they could by magic or intuition have a good understanding of everything each patient needed to know. But relationships like this take effort to form. It may also be difficult for women to give midwives an understanding of what they need to know until they know it. Although it respects autonomy best if information is tailored to the individual needs of women, midwives also need some professional consensus on what the *minimum* amount of information should be. This minimum need not include everything any person could possibly want to know to make a decision, but might be set at a level where the patient knows enough to ask questions that enable the midwife to tailor the rest of the information to the patient's needs. A professional consensus would enable midwives to pool their expertise, professional and personal experience. The danger of this approach is that rather than enhancing the autonomy of patients, it could promote a check-list mentality towards consent, with the minimum quickly becoming the norm. To some extent this has already happened with patient information sheets (PIS). The PIS provides a patient with written (or audio) information that can be taken away and mulled over, but it should not be used as a substitute for conversation or discussion of the relevant information for this gives midwives an opportunity to get to know their patients better and bring to bear their skills of determining what further information would be helpful. The PIS is, though, a tangible record of information that has been imparted, and it is easy to see how with all the pressures on time and resources, a practice of expecting women to initiate any further discussion can develop.

Finally, the timing of the information is important in midwifery. In some respects timing is beyond the control of the midwife. In an ideal world everyone, not just women, would consider issues related to antenatal testing and termination in advance of a pregnancy; indeed, in an ideal world everyone would think about the implications of being pregnant before they became pregnant. Even so, making decisions about termination is likely to be different when one is actually pregnant as opposed to in the abstract, and different also from pregnancy to pregnancy. Decisions about terminating a pregnancy may require women to assimilate unfamiliar information in emotionally charged circumstances. Opinions vary about how much information women should be given as part of consent to antenatal screening tests. Women are certainly not counselled to the same degree about the implications of screening as they are if a test suggests some fetal abnormality. One reason for this is that there are so many different impairments that could be detected, each with its own different prognosis for survival and quality of life; another reason is that a balance has to be struck between the interests of the minority and the interests of the majority. In the majority of cases there will be no detectable impairment and the expense (in its widest sense including stress and anxiety as well as financial resources) of the extensive counselling may be thought to outweigh the harm that comes to the minority of women whose babies are found to have an impairment and who did not really feel adequately prepared for this result.

Things are somewhat different when it comes to discussing the delivery, as birth is an inevitable outcome rather than a statistically remote possibility. It is generally accepted that women should have some genuine choices about the kind of birth they would ideally like. But for these choices to be realistically available, they may have to be made in advance, both to enable service providers to put plans in place that accommodate their choices and for women to make considered and informed judgements about their preferred mode of care. Some decisions cannot be made in advance because it is not possible to predict with certainty what will happen on the day. Other decisions, such as what, if any, pain relief to accept, can be thought about in advance but do not have to be decided in advance. The benefits of giving this information before it is needed are obvious: being in labour is not the best circumstance in which to try to absorb new and unfamiliar information. Indeed, giving information in advance of delivery is current good practice. The problems that may arise when decisions are made in advance will be discussed shortly.

Competence

The starting point for consent is actually competence (sometimes called capacity). It is because one is competent to make the decision for oneself that one should be sufficiently informed and then permitted to make the choice. It is a moot point whether competence and autonomy are synonymous. One has to be competent to be autonomous. Someone who is potentially autonomous can be deceived and misinformed; someone who is potentially autonomous can be coerced to do something against his or her will; but someone who is intrinsically or temporarily incompetent cannot be autonomous. However, being competent to make a particular decision is not the same as being autonomous. Autonomy in philosophy is a much broader concept than competence is in law.

A distinction can also be drawn between being incompetent and being irrational. Autonomous beings can take huge risks autonomously, provided that they understand the nature of those risks. Indeed, it is the ability to understand the nature of the risk that is central, rather than the ability to persuade a third party of the merits of risk-taking. There is a significant difference between accepting that someone is competent and agreeing with the decisions that they make for themselves. Unfortunately, some practitioners—and this comment is not aimed specifically at midwives—seem to generate a faulty kind of syllogism to overcome this difference. It runs something like this:

> I am the expert in this field.
> You would be crazy to ignore my advice.
> You have ignored my advice.
> Therefore you are crazy.
> You are crazy.
> Therefore you are incompetent to make decisions for yourself.
> I am therefore justified in ignoring your incompetent wishes.

Competence is not an absolute state, although incompetence might be. Generally one's competence is relative to what one is being asked to do. You are competent to deliver a baby, I am not, but this does not mean that if I am your patient I am incapable of consenting to the way in which my delivery is managed. In the context of consent, competence means that one understands that one is being required to make a decision about oneself and one understands the information that has to be weighed in the balance to arrive at a decision. Effectively, one also has to be in a position to express the result of this decision since if one is competent but unable (perhaps due to paralysis) to communicate, for the practical purposes of those trying to gain consent, one is rendered incompetent. Likewise, one might be competent to understand the relevant information but be rendered incompetent by the ineffective communication skills of the practitioner attempting to give this information. One can also be rendered incompetent when one does not speak the same language as one's care-giver. It might also be that one is competent to form some kinds of judgement but not others because they are essentially more complex. This is not an observation unique to health care. It has been suggested on many occasions that ordinary jurors are simply unable to grasp the complexities of some fraud cases and that they are therefore incompetent to make a judgement about the guilt or innocence of the defendant.

One should resist the temptation to think in terms of *groups* of individuals being incompetent. In most cases this way of thinking fails to account for the range of abilities within any group and it also fails to recognise that individuals are rarely incompetent per se. Rather they will be competent to make some decisions but not others. It is now being recognised, for instance, that children should not be assumed to be incompetent. Likewise that those with a mental disability are capable of consenting to some things, even quite complex things, if these are explained skilfully enough. However, babies and those who are unconscious are unable, for the time being at least, to make any of their own decisions.

For midwives, any general tendency to identify groups of incompetent patients is particularly fraught with ethical danger since one such group to be defined as incompetent has been women in labour. This is both because it is a painful process and because some of the drugs given to relieve pain can impair a patient's judgement. Against this it can be argued, pretty obviously, that labour comes in various stages, the pain varies from woman to woman, and some forms of pain relief interfere with judgement less than others and affect different people in different ways. So, while some women may become temporarily incompetent during periods of their confinement, few women are incompetent throughout the whole process of childbirth.

It is not uncommon, for the reasons discussed in the previous section, for women to make birth plans prior to their confinement. These can be perceived as consent or refusal of consent—in writing. If birth plans are awarded the status of advance directives this can generate problems if the woman changes her mind during labour, especially if she has told her birth attendant and/or accompanying friend to disregard anything she says in contradiction of her birth plan once labour is underway.

As Ekman Ladd points out, however, some of the consent forms (particularly in the USA) which women sign are not like other consent forms, living wills or advanced directives because labouring women do not have the same 'escape hatches' (Ekman Ladd 1992 p 218) as other patients. If one signs a consent form prior to elective surgery one can always discharge oneself from hospital prior to being given the pre-med, and if one consents to be involved in clinical research one can withdraw at any time from the trial. Moreover, as she says, if one signs an advance directive one can always rip it up if one changes one's mind—it does not come into force until one is incompetent. I agree with Ekman Ladd that since labour is an unavoidable and inevitable outcome of pregnancy one cannot just decide not to go through with the birth after all and leave the hospital. I also accept that in the USA where signing an all encompassing consent form may be a prerequisite to being accepted into the care of a hospital consultant, many women have little choice but to sign and little room for manoeuvre having signed. However, in the UK I do not think that the birth plan drawn up with the midwife is, or should be, granted absolute status. As with an advance directive, the woman can change her mind at any time before labour and expect her new wishes to be given equal respect. I do grant, though, that labouring women are in a more difficult position because of the general tendency to assume they are in too much pain and too afraid to make competent decisions. I also grant that some women may be in agony when they change their mind about an epidural for instance—but what an excellent and completely understandable reason to change one's mind! I likewise think that if someone in such pain is able to continue to refuse an epidural then, because they are refusing in the light of such pain, this is a good reason to respect their sincerity. It is unreasonable of pregnant women or their attendants to try to agree on precisely how a delivery will be managed—down to the last injection or whiff of gas. Each delivery is different and until it is happening it is not possible to predict how it will feel—there are too many variables.

Possibly, part of the problem of consent in this context is that too much emphasis is placed on making contracts prior to the event and too little on women being able to consent while in labour. In this respect, there is a huge difference between expressing a preference and actually contracting to do something. While I might agree with my friend that, for her, a birth without pain relief seems desirable, I would not agree to forcibly prevent anyone giving her pain relief if she found that she could not bear it at the time. The process of gaining consent prior to labour should be a process of counselling and an exchange of information, rather than a contract. The aim should be to facilitate discussion of what can reasonably be expected to happen in a variety of circumstances.

This process of understanding and negotiation should be, and probably is, the norm in modern midwifery practice. There will, however, be occasions where a woman will absolutely insist on a contractual kind of refusal of consent—for instance to a blood transfusion if she is a Jehovah's Witness. Such cases will be dealt with later as ones of conflicts of interest rather than as a problem with competence as such, since it is already well established that a patient, even a pregnant one, who refuses such therapy when competent cannot be given it when she is no longer competent simply because she is now unable to object.

Decision

There is a difference between making a decision and acquiescing. Decision-making is a conscious process whereas to acquiesce is to agree without reflection. Acquiescing is also different to the conscious choice of allowing another to make the decision. Making a decision is the final stage in the process of giving consent; it is also the final point in the process of refusing consent. A refusal of consent should have the same validity as consent. Understandably, when a patient refuses to do something that her carer thinks is in her best interests, her decision is more likely to be questioned than if consent is forthcoming. But if the patient was competent to consent, then she was equally competent to refuse consent. A midwife who was happy to give a procedure on the grounds that consent was received, should be equally comfortable accepting that the procedure cannot now go ahead; unless, of course, it can be shown that a greater degree of competence is required to oppose a professional recommendation than to accept it. Many practitioners seem happy to perform procedures provided their patients simply acquiesce, but this is not obvious until a situation arises where a similar patient refuses to consent.

An argument can be made for applying stricter criteria to refusal to accept expert advice, provided it can be shown that the refusal fundamentally alters the gravity of the decision. This is an argument that is sometimes applied when a patient is refusing a life saving therapy. Buchanan & Brock (1989) suggest that the greater the risks being taken, the greater the need to examine the capacity for a competent decision. This, they claim, accords not only with the law but also common sense. We would, for instance, be prepared to let a child determine what he or she ate for lunch, but not whether and where to invest huge sums of money (Buchanan & Brock 1989). It is not, however, clear why it is risk per se that makes all the difference rather than simply the complexity of the decision required. This point is made by Wicclair (1991) when he modifies the lunch example by asking us to suppose that the child's choice will actually produce a violent allergic reaction in that child. It is not the risk of the violent reaction which renders the child unable to choose, but rather doubts about whether the child understands what a violent allergic reaction is. If the child does not understand, then it is not a matter of being paternalistic when choosing his or her lunch, but rather it is a case of making a proxy decision. Thus, when determining the validity of a patient's refusal of consent, a minimum *competence* test (which varies according to the complexity of the decision) provides greater protection to patient autonomy than a minimum *risk* test, though the latter may provide better protection for the patient from harm as perceived by others.

PATERNALISM AND PROXY DECISIONS

Paternalism occurs when someone's capacity to make their own decision is ignored. It can take the form of overriding an actual decision, not bothering to get a decision in the first place, or deliberately manipulating a decision by misleading the patient through the information given or withheld. Employing any of these techniques invalidates consent and renders the procedure concerned involuntary. A clear distinction needs to be made between 'involuntary' and 'nonvoluntary'. The latter concerns action taken without the patient's consent because the patient is incompetent to consent. Paternalism occurs when a procedure is carried out involuntarily. Where an action is nonvoluntary it results from a proxy or surrogate decision, not paternalism.

Paternalism and proxy decision-making are easily confused because, however misguided, paternalism is essentially benevolent. Someone acting paternalistically is motivated by the desire to do the best for the subject of their attention, just like those who make proxy decisions. The difference is that whereas the subject of the proxy decision is incapable of making a choice, the paternalist considers that they know better than the subject where the subject's best interests lie, even though the subject is capable of deciding for him or herself. So, to perform an episiotomy against a woman's wishes because one envisages extensive tearing, is paternalistic. To decide to perform an episiotomy while the woman is delirious (and thereby incompetent) from pain and analgesics is to make a proxy decision. These distinctions can be made without judging either one to be the correct or the wrong response. The road to hell may be paved with good intentions, but even so there is a significant difference between actions that are motivated by benevolence and those that are performed indifferently, out of self-interest, or even maliciously.

There is considerable debate over who is best placed to act as proxy—particularly for small children. In the labour suite, the same kind of debate may occur between the doctor, midwife and accompanying partner or friend of the patient, each of whom can make a strong case for being the one to decide on an incompetent patient's behalf. One difference between children and pregnant women in this regard is that pregnant women can actually specify in advance whose judgement they wish to take precedence. Practitioners are unlikely to find this a problem when it is they who the patient designates but if it is the friend, hostility may result. Nevertheless, in ethical terms, provided that the patient specified that the friend act as the proxy, then if the patient's autonomy must be respected so should the decisions of her designated proxy.

It is possible that the attempt to reject the patient's appointed proxy by the professional practitioner is an indication of a deeper problem than simply that of determining who is in the best position to decide on the patient's behalf. Anyone's commitment to the principle of respect for autonomy would be severely tested in circumstances where a patient is slowly dying because the proxy is refusing some procedure like a blood transfusion. Refusing to acknowledge the status of a proxy enables carers to avoid the issue of the extent to which we are free to make decisions that might result in our being seriously harmed. This leads us to a series of specific questions about the limits that can be legitimately placed on a patient's autonomy.

LIMITS TO AUTONOMY

Can a woman bring harm on herself?

In order to avoid duplicating material covered earlier, in this section the specific question of whether one can autonomously harm oneself, and if so, in what circumstances will be discussed.

It is clear that our autonomous choices are not restricted to acting only in our own interests—at least not if these are narrowly defined. We frequently do things that we might otherwise not do when asked by someone we love. We devote more time to work than we are strictly paid to do when someone needs us or to help out a colleague. Many of us who are parents would willingly sacrifice our lives to save those of our children. Such examples illustrate the sense in which we autonomously choose to limit our actions in ways that do not apparently directly advantage us. Clearly it could be argued that really we are not harmed by so doing because it serves our longer-term interests in some kind of you-scratch-my-back-I'll-scratch-yours social contract sense. But what about the decision to die for our children?

Here it is not so clear that our long-term interests are served since we will no longer be around to reap the benefits.

In this case, it is not that our wider interests are served but rather that there are at least some things that we value more than ourselves—the lives of our children perhaps. There are other things that people have been willing to die for too—their religious or political beliefs for example. In such cases, even though we do not necessarily share the views of those willing to make this sacrifice, we often do accept that they should be free to make such choices and we do not always find such decisions to be irrational. The extent to which we find them irrational depends in large measure on whether we think that the end of the action is actually something inherently more valuable than life.

It seems, then, that a substantial part of our willingness to accept the self-harming actions of patients will flow from the coherence to us of the justification that they give for their actions. The danger of using this as the sole basis of determining whether or not patients should be free to make their own decisions is that it is an invitation for unlimited paternalism with patients only being given the freedom to choose what would in any case have been chosen for them. We must be in a position to determine whether the difference of judgement here turns on some kind of faulty decision-making capacity of the patient, or whether the disagreement is essentially one between different values. For this reason, we need a fairly rigorous but tolerant notion of what constitutes coherent justification.

One aspect of coherent justification for an action would be to consider whether or not the decision was consistent with the values the patient claimed to hold: to ask, does it facilitate the state of affairs that the patient desires, or hinder it? In this sense, the decision being made could be said to reflect the patient's true self.

Even if one is assured that the patient's decision-making faculty is not impaired, one might still wonder whether the decision has been made autonomously, for one might question whether the values that underpin the decision were actually autonomously chosen. Many of our values reflect social conditioning, family influence and so forth and do not result from considered reflection. Since, however, this is true of so many of us, is it reasonable to expect patients refusing intervention to be able to justify the values that they hold better than other people, or indeed patients complying with treatment recommendations? Equally, it is also necessary to recognise instances where there is more reason to question the autonomous decision to hold the values.

There is a legal judgement in one such case. A pregnant woman was admitted to hospital accompanied by her mother, who was a Jehovah's Witness. After her mother had left home the daughter had been raised by her father, who was not a Witness. At the time of admission to hospital, there was no reason to suppose that a blood transfusion would be necessary. However, after being alone for several hours with her mother, the daughter mentioned to a nurse that she would not wish to be given a blood transfusion should it become necessary to have one. Unfortunately, following the birth of a still-born baby by caesarean section, a transfusion was indicated but the staff were reluctant to give one since the daughter was both an adult and had appeared competent at the time her instruction was issued. Her father was incensed, convinced that the mother had taken the opportunity to brainwash their daughter while she was vulnerable and susceptible to persuasion. He successfully petitioned for the blood to be given. Here the issue was not one of whether religious views should be accepted, whatever the consequences for the believer, but rather whether the supposed believer freely held the religious views she used to justify her decision (*Re T* 1992).

Can a woman make decisions the effects of which bring harm to the fetus?

This discussion will be limited to the actions of women who intend to take their pregnancies to term. Excluded, then, is the decision to have a termination of pregnancy, which is clearly the most common decision made by women that could be said to harm the fetus.

It is generally held that while we are free to bring harm on ourselves, we are not free to bring harm on others. This is not, however, an absolute rule since it is applied under a presumption in favour of autonomy. This means that some harm to others is tolerated where this harm is minor and the cost of preventing it in terms of individual liberty would be great. Our autonomy would be virtually worthless if this were not so, since almost any action we take has harmful side-effects on someone. Taking the train might be less damaging to the environment, but that does not mean that no damage to the environment is caused by trains. However, the more serious the harm, the more likely we are to expect a sacrifice of individual freedom to avoid it.

The difficulty with applying this general principle in the case of pregnant women is that in attempting to resolve the competing interests—the fetus's interest in not being harmed and the woman's interest in her autonomy—we recognise that avoiding harm to the fetus can require much more of an imposition on the woman than avoiding harm generally requires. It may require an actual bodily intrusion, like a caesarean section, keyhole surgery or the taking of some drug. At the other end of the spectrum, it might entail some behaviour modification, and somewhere in the middle, interference with the woman's views about the mode of her confinement that may, in some circumstances, compromise her ideals.

One way of analysing this problem is to see it as a conflict between maternal and fetal rights—the woman's rights over her own body versus the fetus's right not to be harmed. Into this conflict, people then bring their views about the status of the fetus (either comparing it to any other person and awarding strong claims in terms of its interests, or holding that it has no claims either due to its gestational development or due to its dependence on and location within its mother's body). Also, they bring their views about the obligations of the pregnant woman, some holding that women who are pregnant have special obligations to their fetus by virtue of choosing to go ahead with the pregnancy, others that the obligations are no different to those that could be expected of any other person whose liberty was being curtailed to a similar degree.

There is not space here to flesh out this rather intractable debate. My own position is that at least *some* pregnant women do have special obligations to their fetus(es). This is not by virtue of having chosen to continue with the pregnancy per se, but by virtue of having taken on the mantle of motherhood (which is not something all pregnant women have done—an obvious example here would be a woman acting as a surrogate).

The possibilities afforded by modern technology have resulted in a debate about the true nature of motherhood, posing questions such as whether motherhood is based on genetic relationships, bearing a baby or rearing a child. Perhaps motherhood can more accurately be defined in terms of a moral relationship, where a woman takes on certain moral obligations towards a particular child. If this is so, then the very least such an obligation would entail is that of care and nurture. In this case, a mother might be obliged to accept more of an infringement of her liberties for the protection of her child than another person might be expected to endure for the protection of someone else's child or a stranger. This does not mean that pregnant mothers are obliged to do anything, no matter how serious the consequences for themselves, for the benefit of the fetus. Instead, it means that mothers would be obliged to undertake major infringements of liberty where it can be shown that this would definitely be of major benefit to the fetus. The less definite the benefit, or the less the benefit, the less sacrifice mothers are obliged to make, although a minor sacrifice for a small benefit might also be required. Women who have chosen to continue with a pregnancy for reasons other than to be mothers, do have obligations to consider the interests of the future child, but this is not a special obligation. Rather it is on a par with the obligations generally placed on any of us not to cause unnecessary harm. Such a general obligation may require significantly less self-sacrifice than that placed on mothers, or so it could be argued.

Here, I am relying on mothers to moderate their own behaviour according to their own beliefs about what is in the best interests of their child. Quite a different set of arguments would be needed to compel mothers to make these sacrifices. The very least such a justification would require is that either all parents (both fathers and mothers) should be prepared so to sacrifice, or that all people would be prepared so to sacrifice, even for strangers. This is a view that I have developed elsewhere (Draper 1996).

Having a coherent ethical justification for non-interference in a pregnant woman's autonomous decision, even though this will cause irreparable damage to the fetus, will be cold comfort to the midwives involved. The lesson to be learned from these situations is that there is an ethical, as well as a pragmatic, need to negotiate with pregnant women before emergencies arise. If it is the case that women enter pregnancies with certain expectations about the care that they will receive and also presuming that nothing will go wrong for them, this is perhaps the fault of the health care professionals who have, in the past, promised more than they are able to deliver. If labouring women are distrustful of the advice that they are given, this is perhaps because so many procedures have been given for spurious clinical reasons or for the convenience of practitioners. Just as there are good grounds for arguing that mothers have to take their ethical responsibilities for their fetuses seriously, professionals can also be charged with obligations to ensure that the information they give to women as part of gaining consent is true, based on sound research, and up to date.

References

Buchanan A E, Brock D W 1989 Deciding for others. Cambridge University Press, Cambridge

Draper H 1996 Women, forced caesareans and antenatal responsibilities. Journal of Medical Ethics 22:327–333

Ekman Ladd R 1992 Women in labour: some issues in informed consent. In: Holmes H B, Purdy L M (eds) Feminist perspectives in medical ethics. Indiana University Press, Bloomington

Gillon R 1986 Philosophical medical ethics. Wiley, Chichester

Re T 1992 4 All England Law Reports 649

Royal College of Midwives 2002 Position paper 25 home births. Online. Available: www.rem.org.uk

Wicclair M R 1991 Patient decision making: capacity and risk. Bioethics 15:91–104

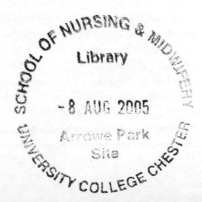

Chapter 2

Legal and ethical issues in midwifery practice

Jean V. McHale

INTRODUCTION

Pregnancy gives rise to a host of ethical and legal dilemmas concerning the status of mother and fetus. Women have the right to make choices during pregnancy and the right to choose has been bolstered in a series of guidelines such as the Department of Health document *Changing Childbirth* in 1994 (DoH 1994). This document stressed the need for respect for maternal choice during pregnancy and birth. The report noted three principles: first, that the woman should be the focus of maternity care provision, second, that maternity services should be readily accessible to all and third, that services provided should be both effective and efficient. While this document provides a rhetorical backdrop to the current practice, what choices do pregnant women have and what constraints on their choices during pregnancy can be imposed? This chapter explores some of the many and varied legal and ethical dilemmas that arise from midwifery practice, both in the hospital setting and in the community. It considers first pregnancy, then the birth and finally the issue of postnatal care. The role of the law in this area in the future is likely to be further influenced by the operation of the Human Rights Act 1998. This legislation enables the court to take account of the provisions of the European Convention on Human Rights and case law from the European Court of Human Rights. A number of the Convention rights may be particularly applicable here, notably Article 2—the right to life, Article 3—the right not to be subject to torture or inhuman or degrading treatment, and Article 8—the right to privacy. Various aspects of these rights are considered below.

PREGNANCY

Research has made us increasingly aware of the impact that maternal behaviour during pregnancy may have on the health of the infant and this has led to health promotion campaigns encouraging healthy behaviour during pregnancy.

The midwife can play an important role in the provision of information regarding good care during pregnancy, but how far can and should this go? Fundamentally the mother does have autonomy over how she behaves during pregnancy. An attempt to physically restrain her may give rise to liability in civil law for the tort of battery arising from unlawful touching or for one of the criminal law offences such as common law assault and battery (see McHale 2002b). The law goes further and does not allow legal proceedings to be brought on behalf of the fetus which would restrict the mother's own autonomy. In *Re F* (*in utero*) ([1988] 2 All ER 193) a local authority sought to have a fetus made a ward of court. The local authority was concerned about the welfare of the fetus due to the nomadic lifestyle of the mother who had a history of drug abuse and mental illness. The Court of Appeal rejected this application confirming the approach in earlier cases, notably that of *Paton v BPAS* ([1978] 2 All ER 987). In that case Sir George Baker had held that

> The foetus cannot in English law, in my view have any right of its
> own at least until it is born and has a separate existence from its
> mother. That permeates the whole of the civil law of this country ...
> and is indeed the basis of the decisions in those countries where law
> is founded on the common law, that is today in America, Canada,
> Australia and I have no doubt in others.

In *Re F* the Court of Appeal noted that the effect of the order that was being sought in that case would be to enable the mother's actions to be subject to control. Balcolme LJ, with whom the other members of the Court of Appeal agreed, stated that

> If Parliament were to think it appropriate that a pregnant woman
> should be subject to controls for the benefit of her unborn child,

then doubtless it will stipulate the circumstances in which such controls may be applied and the safeguards appropriate for the mother's protection. In such a sensitive field, affecting as it does the liberty of the individual, it is not for the judiciary to extend the law.

(The statement in *Paton* has been supported in a series of later cases e.g. *Re MB*—discussed later—and *AG Reference (No 3 of 1994)* [1997] 3 WLR 421).

There is a remote possibility that, where a woman is reckless during pregnancy and the consequence of her behaviour is that she miscarries, a prosecution for manslaughter might result (Fovargue & Miola 1998) or that there might be a prosecution under the Infant Life Preservation Act 1929 which makes it an offence to destroy the life of a child that is capable of being born alive. However bringing such an action would in practice be very difficult (Glazebrook 1993, Kennedy 1991). In relation to actions for damages in civil law, again legal proceedings are problematic and the prospect for successful litigation is limited. The Congenital Disabilities and Civil Liability Act 1976 does not allow a woman to be sued by her child where her behaviour results in harm being caused to the fetus during pregnancy.[1] An exception exists in relation to injuries caused when driving a car. The reason for the exception here is that in practice a negligence action is being brought against the woman's insurers rather than against the woman herself. Liability under the Act may however arise if there is a duty owed to the mother, for example, to warn her of particular risks that she faces during pregnancy, and that duty is broken and harm results to the fetus. We return to this issue next.

The approach of English law in this area is in sharp contrast to the interventionist approach that has been taken in the USA. There was a period from the mid-1970s until the early 1990s in certain US states when the law was used to compel behaviour by many pregnant women, such as receiving blood transfusions, or to subject them to sanctions for behaving in a manner that was harmful to the fetus during pregnancy. Where a stillbirth had resulted allegedly due to the woman's conduct, there were resulting prosecutions for charges such as fetal drug delivery, fetal abuse or manslaughter (Bewley 2002, Daniels 2002, Robertson 1994, Savage 2002). Such

---

[1] Note that the position prior to when the Act came into force in 1976 is governed by common law and in such a situation there may be a duty in common law to the fetus (*Burton v Islington HA* [1992] 3 All ER 833 CA). However, in practice, due to the operation of limitation periods regarding negligence actions the prospect for such actions is reducing over time.

direct legal measures were accompanied by a very active campaign of social education. Again in the USA warnings against consumption during pregnancy were common on alcohol containers and cigarette packets. There are acute tensions as commentators such as Bewley (2002) have noted. In her discussion of the prospects for restraining the pregnant drug taker, she highlights the tensions between what might be regarded as the moral obligation of the pregnant woman (namely to take reasonable steps to ensure that the fetus is born in good health) and the wish of society to reduce harmful maternal behaviour during pregnancy. She persuasively argues that a strategy of threats is not only morally undesirable but also there is no medical evidence that adequately supports its operation.

In legal terms any attempt to impose any restraints on the pregnant woman in the UK can be seen as particularly problematic in the light of the Human Rights Act 1998. This legislation enables English courts to interpret existing law—whether case or statute law—in the light of the European Convention of Human Rights and to make reference to the case law of the European Court of Human Rights. Any attempt to impose restraints on a pregnant woman in such a situation may be regarded as a violation of Article 3 of the European Convention of Human Rights, which prohibits the imposition of inhuman or degrading treatment; and also of her rights under Article 8, which grants a right to privacy that may be interpreted to encompass autonomy of action (Wicks 2001). In *X and Y v Netherlands* ((1986) 8 EHRR 235) it was stated that private life relates to a person's physical integrity. Some, however, might seek to argue that restraints on women are legitimated in the interests of the fetus and in particular in the light of the right to life of the fetus, which is arguably supported by Article 2—the right to life. However, as we shall see, while this argument may be advanced, sustaining it may be problematic in view of the somewhat ambivalent approach taken in the past to the status of the fetus at the European Court of Human Rights.

Women have access to a wide range of tests during pregnancy that provide them with information about the progress of the pregnancy from dating scans to any potential problems that might arise, for example in relation to fetal health. Tests undertaken during pregnancy may give rise to a whole host of ethical and legal dilemmas (Alderson 2002). A controversial issue is the use of HIV testing during pregnancy. Such tests are voluntary and to undertake a test without consent will almost certainly give rise to liability in battery. Nonetheless the reality of free voluntary testing has been questioned (de Zulueta 2002). For example, guidelines such as those of the UK

Intercollegiate Working Party (1998) have emphasised the need for a directive approach, which would arguably undermine the reality of the consent process. (This issue is explored further in Chapter 4.) Controversy has also surrounded the issue of whether the sex of the fetus should be disclosed to parents, where scans have been undertaken, because of the emphasis placed in some cultures on the importance of bearing male children. There are some hospitals in the UK where, in the light of concerns regarding sex selection, health care professionals are not prepared to reveal the sex of the fetus. If a test reveals a potential problem that may be remedied by clinical intervention during pregnancy with the mother's consent, then no difficulties arise. In practice, however, there is currently only a very limited prospect of any effective medical intervention as a consequence of screening. Some women may wish to avail themselves of information regarding antenatal testing, go ahead with screening and then, if the fetus is found to be impaired or to be at risk of developing an impairment after birth, consider the prospect of an abortion.

Abortion itself is unlawful under the Offences Against the Person Act 1861 section 58, which makes it an offence to unlawfully procure a miscarriage, and the Infant Life Preservation Act 1929 section 1(1), which provides that it is an offence to destroy the life of a child capable of being born alive. However the Abortion Act 1967 (as amended) allows abortions to be undertaken where the criteria that are set out in the Act have been satisfied. The 1967 Act does not provide a woman with a right to an abortion. Instead two doctors must be satisfied that the criteria established in the legislation are complied with (although in an emergency one doctor is sufficient). First, where continuation of the pregnancy would result in greater risk to the physical and mental health of the woman than if the pregnancy were terminated (s1(1)(a)). Under this subsection abortions can be performed up to the 24th week of pregnancy. It can be argued that abortion on the basis of sex selection may fall within this category (for further discussion of this area see Morgan 1988). Second, an abortion may be obtained where the termination is necessary to prevent grave permanent injury to the health of the woman or her family (s1(1)(b)); and third, where continuing the pregnancy would involve a risk to the life of the woman which was greater than if the pregnancy were terminated (s1(1)(c)). Finally, and arguably particularly relevant in this context, is section 1(1)(d), which sanctions abortion up until birth in the situation where there is a substantial risk that were the child to be born he or she would be seriously handicapped. The nature and the extent of this provision is riven with uncertainty

(Morgan 1990, Sheldon and Wilkinson 2001). While it encompasses severe physical and mental disability that would manifest itself at birth, it is unclear to what extent it would apply to a condition that may arise several years or even decades later but then manifest itself as a serious degenerative disorder. This is an issue that will become ever more pertinent as the scope and range of genetic testing during pregnancy increases still further. Again the approach taken under the Abortion Act 1967 itself may be the subject of challenge in the courts under the Human Rights Act 1998 in the context of the application of Article 2 of the European Convention of Human Rights that sets out the right to life (see below, p 48).

There is a further issue that arises; namely, what if the testing undertaken during pregnancy itself goes wrong and injury to the fetus results? English law does not enable a child to bring what is known as a wrongful life action on the basis that he or she should not have been born (*McKay v Essex HA* [1982] 1 QB 1166). An action may, however, be brought by the parents for the distress caused. Where a live baby results who is disabled, contrary to tests undertaken, this may lead to an action being brought for negligence. The parents may claim compensation under a wrongful birth action on the basis that had they been told of the consequences the pregnancy would have been terminated. In addition there is the possibility that proceedings may be brought in a situation in which the pregnancy was terminated and the information given to the woman leading to her decision to terminate was incorrect (Montgomery 2002).

DELIVERY AND BIRTH

While women have in theory a much broader range of delivery methods in practice such choice may be somewhat limited. For example, as Montgomery (2002) has commented, the Department of Health Maternity Services Charter 'falls short of promising women the right to home births instead giving women the right to information "as to where they can give birth"'. There is no right to demand access to a particular clinical procedure/resources simply because one regards this as preferable. Traditionally the courts have also been unwilling to intervene in resource allocation decisions by NHS bodies (see, for instance, *R v Cambridge District Health Authority ex parte B* [1995] 2 All ER 129).

When it arises, however, how does the law regulate a situation where the clinical team believe that clinical intervention is appropriate and the woman resists and wants to have a different approach?

As noted above, English law gives a woman a right to consent and to refuse consent to clinical procedures. This was confirmed in *Re T* ([1992] 4 All ER 649). However in this case Lord Donaldson, while confirming the right to refuse, inserted one caveat. He stated that

> An adult patient who suffers from no mental incapacity, has an absolute right to choose one rather than another of the treatments being offered. The only possible qualification is a case in which the choice may lead to the death of a viable foetus ... if and when [such a case] arises the court will be faced with a novel problem of considerable ethical and legal complexity.

In a series of subsequent cases the English courts were faced with a conflict between a woman who was refusing medical procedures including a caesarean section and the clinical team who thought that clinical intervention was necessary. In *Re S* ([1992] 4 All ER 671) S was 6 days overdue and a caesarean section was proposed because the fetus was in transverse lie. S, a born again Christian, opposed the procedure as she would have required a blood transfusion, which she stated to be contrary to her religious beliefs. The hospital sought a declaration that the procedure was lawful and this was granted by Sir Stephen Brown. This is a controversial case that relied on a US case *Re AC* ([1990] 573 A. 2d 1235) that itself did not provide strong support for the finding. The judgement here was also very brief. *Re S* was subject to considerable criticism both from academic commentators and from health care professional bodies. The Royal College of Obstetricians and Gynaecologists (RCOG) issued guidelines to the effect that the imposition of a caesarean section on a pregnant woman would be unethical (RCOG 1994). Nevertheless, caesarean sections were sanctioned in a number of subsequent cases with, in some instances, women being sectioned under the Mental Health Act 1983 in order that the section could be undertaken (*Tameside v Glossop* [1996] 1 FCR 753, *Rochdale NHS Trust v C* [1997] 1 FCR 274 and *Norfolk & Norwich NHS Trust v W* [1996] 2 FLR 613). Finally, however, in *Re MB* the Court of Appeal firmly rejected such an approach. She was held to be incompetent and the caesarean section was authorised. Here Butler Sloss LJ held that.

> A competent woman who has the capacity to decide may, for religious reasons, other reasons, for rational or irrational reasons or for no reason at all, choose not to have medical intervention, even though the consequence may be the death or serious handicap of the child she bears, or her own death. In that event the courts do not have the jurisdiction to declare medical intervention lawful and the question of her own best interests objectively considered, does not arise.

The Court of Appeal confirmed earlier decisions such as *Paton v BPAS* ([1978] 2 All ER 987). One issue was a perceived inconsistency between the safeguards given to the fetus from termination save in very exceptional circumstances late in pregnancy, and the decision which was being reached in this particular case to refuse to sanction a caesarean section. However, Butler Sloss LJ commented that

> Although it may seem illogical that a child capable of being born alive is protected by the criminal law from intentional destruction, and by the Abortion Act from termination otherwise than as permitted by the Act, but is not protected from the [irrational] decision of a competent mother not to allow medical intervention to avert the risk of death, this appears to be the present state of the law.

The Court of Appeal's approach was followed in *St George's NHS Trust v S* ([1998] 3 All ER 673). In this case the court condemned the use of the Mental Health Act 1983 to detain a woman for the purposes of then sanctioning a caesarean section on her without her consent. In this case the woman was sectioned, the caesarean was undertaken and the woman was then promptly released. Judge LJ held

> When human life is at stake the pressure to provide an affirmative answer authorising unwarranted medical intervention is very powerful. Nevertheless, the autonomy of each individual requires continuing protection even, perhaps particularly, when the motive for interfering with it is readily understandable and indeed to many would appear commendable.

The enforced caesarean cases have been the subject of considerable academic debate (Bailey Harris 1998, McHale 2002b, Wells 1998). The perceived tensions between the abortion restrictions and the right of refusal sanctioned in this particular case have been noted. So too has the fact that the decision in this case concerned the right of a competent woman to refuse. The difficulty that arises is in the determination of competence in a particular situation. In *Re MB* itself the Court of Appeal followed the test for competence which was set out in an earlier decision that of *Re C* ([1994] 1 All ER 649) and the recommendations set out in the Law Commission's Report on Mental Incapacity (Law Commission 1995). They set out the test of capacity accordingly:

> … a person lacks capacity to make a decision where
>
> (a) the person is unable to comprehend and retain the information which is material to the decision, especially as to the likely consequences of having or not having the treatment in question: and

(b) the patient is unable to use the information and weigh it in the balance as of the process of arriving at a decision.

One concern expressed by academic commentators is that while the Court of Appeal in *Re MB* adhered to the principle of respect for the individual's autonomy, there is still potential for autonomy to be undermined in practice. This is of concern because English law provides that, in a situation in which an adult is declared incompetent, clinical procedures can be undertaken on the basis of necessity as it is in their best interests (*Re F* [1990] 2 AC 1). Temporary incompetence, as the Court of Appeal commented in *Re MB*, may erode capacity. This may be due to factors, mentioned by Lord Donaldson in the earlier case of *Re T*, such as 'confusion, shock, pain and drugs'. The concept of temporary incompetence was used in *Re MB* to legitimise the performance of the caesarean section in that particular case. The Court of Appeal upheld the decision of the judge in the first instance to the effect that MB lacked capacity. MB was competent to consent to the caesarean section itself, however, she was not competent to refuse the procedure as she was 'at that moment suffering an impairment of her mental functioning which disabled her. She was temporarily incompetent'. The Court found that it was her phobia of needles that impaired her ability to decide.

Given the difficulties surrounding the determination of the boundaries of competence and the consequences for a patient who is declared to be incompetent in *St George's NHS Trust v S*, the Court of Appeal established guidelines that should be followed in subsequent cases in which a patient is refusing therapy. It is important to note that these guidelines do not apply where the woman is competent to consent or to refuse consent. Where it is proposed to perform a caesarean section on a protesting woman this procedure would require the sanction of the High Court. In such a situation the woman should be involved or where she herself was unable to be directly involved, for example, if she was unconscious, the Official Solicitor should represent her. In making its determination the court should consider evidence of competence. It is to be hoped that use of such guidelines will reduce any prospect of the autonomy of the competent woman being undermined in the future.

These cases were decided before the enactment of the Human Rights Act 1998. This legislation now enables, as noted, the English courts to interpret English law in the light of the provisions of the European Convention of Human Rights. Nonetheless it is questionable whether a different approach will be taken. In the past the European Court of Human Rights has been circumspect in its consideration of the position of the fetus. The European Commission on Human Rights, while taking the approach that there is no absolute right to life, has largely left open the issue of the application of Article 2 in relation to the fetus (see e.g. *Paton v UK* (1980) 3 EHRR 408; *Open Door Counselling and Dublin Well Woman v Ireland* (1992) 15 EHRR 244). It has been suggested that because in the context of the European Court of Human Rights states have been afforded a considerable 'margin of appreciation,' the English courts may also be of the view that this is an issue on which a conclusive determination is the provenance of parliament rather than of the courts (Stauch 2001).

A further issue in relation to the delivery occurs when something goes wrong. Is the midwife in such a situation subject to legal liability? In the law of negligence a health care professional may be held liable where a duty of care arises. This applies where it is reasonably foreseeable that the person would be affected by the actions of the defendant. Establishing a prima facie duty in such a situation, whether in the hospital delivery suite or at home in the case of a home birth, would not be difficult. Next it must be established whether the midwife has failed to act in accordance with the standard of care that today is expected of a responsible body of professional practice. In the past as long as there was expert evidence supporting the approach taken by a particular body of professional practice applying, then liability did not arise (*Bolam v Friern Hospital Management Company* [1957] 2 All ER 118). In recent years, however, there have been increasing indications that the judiciary are more willing to take a 'hard look' at the course of action undertaken by the professional body. In the House of Lords, Lord Browne Wilkinson stated that

In particular where there are questions of assessment of the relative risks and benefits of adopting a particular medical practice, a reasonable view necessarily presupposes that the relative risks and benefits have been weighed by the experts in forming their opinions. But if in a rare case, it can be demonstrated that the professional opinion is not capable of withstanding logical analysis, the judge is entitled to hold that the body of opinion is not reasonable or responsible. I emphasise that in my view it will be very seldom right for a judge to reach the conclusion that views genuinely held by a competent medical expert are unreasonable. (*Bolitho v City of Hackney HA* [1988] AC 232)

Since *Bolitho*, as Montgomery notes, the impact of the case has been mixed with the judiciary being more responsive to the hard look approach in *Bolitho* in some cases than others (Montgomery 2002). Nonetheless there are indications from the judiciary that deference to clinical opinion may truly be a thing of the past (Woolf 2001).

POSTNATAL CARE

After birth and, in the case of a hospital birth, after leaving hospital a community midwife will be involved in care of the mother. The law requires that midwives are involved in the care of the mother and infant for the first 10 days after delivery. This period may extend up to 28 days after birth (Nurses, Midwives and Health Visitors Rules 1983 as amended Part V). At this point the health visitor will then take over in the care process. As during the delivery, the midwife is required to seek assistance from a doctor in circumstances that 'deviate from the norm' (rule 40). Usually in such cases care involves practical advice and reassurance being provided to the mother, but there may be situations in which further medical intervention is required. A baby, for example, may have developed jaundice and need to be readmitted to hospital for ultraviolet light treatment. In contrast to the earlier stages in pregnancy the midwife is now dealing with what in law are two patients—mother and child. There may be instances in which the midwife believes that the child requires further therapy and that the parents are being obstructive and indeed are being positively harmful to the welfare of the child in this particular instance. Parents have rights to determine the care of their child. Nonetheless there may be exceptional situations in which it is believed that the welfare of the child is being put at very serious risk. In such circumstances it may be deemed appropriate to seek legal intervention to compel care. In *D v Berkshire CC* ([1987] 1 All ER 20 HL) a registered drug addict gave birth. The child was eventually taken into care after she suffered symptoms of withdrawal and was taken into intensive care. The broader implications of such an approach in terms of maternal constraints have been criticised (Montgomery 1987). It is exceedingly controversial to remove a child from its parents on the basis of what in effect may be regarded as a 'life-style' choice. Nonetheless should the midwife have concerns regarding the care of the child, she may make the decision to inform the relevant manager and this may lead to the issue being referred to the trust solicitors who will determine what in that particular instance is the most appropriate action to take.

Finally, the midwife may be involved in the process of notification of birth. The Births and Deaths Registration Act 1952 provides that the parents are required to register the birth within 42 days. Where the parents have not undertaken this task then any 'qualified informant' shall do so—this is other persons present at the birth or those persons who have care of the child (s1(2)2). The district medical officer is also to be notified of the birth and in practice a doctor or midwife frequently undertakes this task. In the case of stillbirth, which is defined as a situation in which the baby is born dead after the 24th week of pregnancy (Births and Deaths Registration Act 1952 s.41) the legislation also requires that details of the stillbirth shall be registered. In addition in a situation in which there is reason to believe that the child was in fact born alive then the coroner should be informed.

CONCLUSION

Midwifery practice gives rise to some acute ethical and legal dilemmas, as outlined. Professional practice guidelines exhort respect for the autonomy of the woman and this is reflected in English law. The law facilitates maternal choice and provides comparatively few constraints during pregnancy, delivery and postnatal care. Nonetheless there is uncertainty over a range of issues. First, to what extent will genetic screening and the prospect of effective clinical interventions in the womb give rise to further legal challenges and judicial reconsideration of the status of the fetus in English law? Second, will the courts in the future be faced with difficult cases concerning the boundaries of capacity where a pregnant woman decides to refuse a caesarean section? Third, to what extent will the application of the Human Rights Act 1998, and in particular Article 2 the right to life and Article 8 the right to privacy, require us to fundamentally reconsider the legal regulation of the maternal–fetal relationship?

References

Alderson P 2002 Prenatal counselling and images of disability. In: Dickenson D (ed) Ethical issues in maternal-fetal medicine. Cambridge University Press, Cambridge

Bailey Harris R 1998 Pregnancy, autonomy and refusal of medical treatment. Law Quarterly Review 550

Bewley S 2002 Restricting the freedom of pregnant women. In: Dickenson D (ed) Ethical issues in maternal-fetal medicine. Cambridge University Press, Cambridge

Daniels C 2002 Between fathers and fetuses. In: Dickenson D (ed) Ethical issues in maternal-fetal medicine. Cambridge University Press, Cambridge

de Zulueta P 2002 HIV in pregnancy. In: Dickenson D (ed) Ethical issues in maternal-fetal medicine. Cambridge University Press, Cambridge

Department of Health 1994 Changing childbirth. DoH, London

Fovargue S, Miola J 1998 Policing pregnancy: implications of the Attorney-General's reference (No 3 of 1994). Medical Law Review 6:265

Glazebrook P 1993 What care must be taken of an unborn child. Cambridge Law Journal X:20

Kennedy I 1991 A woman and her unborn child. In: Byrne P (ed) Ethics and law in health care and research. Wiley, Chichester

Law Commission 1995 Mental incapacity. HMSO, London

McHale J 2002a A duty not to reproduce? In: Dickenson D (ed) Ethical issues in maternal-fetal medicine. Cambridge University Press, Cambridge

McHale J 2002b Consent and the competent adult patient. In: Tingle J, Cribb A (eds) Nursing law and ethics. Blackwell Scientific, Oxford

Morgan D 1988 Foetal sex identification, abortion and the law. Family Law 355

Morgan D 1990 Abortion; the unexamined ground? Criminal Law Review 687

Montgomery J 1987 Mothers and unborn children. Family Law 227

Montgomery J 2002 Health care law, 2nd edn. Oxford University Press, Oxford

Robertson J 1994 Children of choice. Princeton University Press, Princeton, NJ

Royal College of Obstetricians and Gynaecologists 1994 A consideration of the law and ethics concerning court-ordered obstetric intervention. RCOG, London

Savage W 2002 Caesarean section—who chooses, the woman or her doctor? In: Dickenson D (ed) Ethical issues in maternal-fetal medicine. Cambridge University Press, Cambridge

Sheldon S, Wilkinson S 2001 Termination of pregnancy for reason of foetal disability: are there grounds for a special exception in Law 9. Medical Law Review 85

Stauch M 2001 Pregnancy and the Human Rights Act. In: Garwood-Gowers A, Tingle J, Lewis T (eds) Healthcare Law: the impact of the Human Rights Act 1998. Cavendish, London

Wells C 1998 On the outside looking in: perspectives on enforced caesarians. In: Sheldon S and Thomson M (eds) Feminist perspectives on health care law. Cavendish, London

Wicks E 2001 The right to refuse medical treatment under the European Convention of Human Rights. Medical Law Review 17

Woolf Lord 2001 Are the courts excessively deferential to the medical profession? Medical Law Review 1

UK Intercollegiate Working Party for Enhancing Voluntary Confidential HIV Testing in Pregnancy 1998 Reducing mother to child transmission of HIV infection in the UK. Royal College of Paediatrics and Child Health, London

Chapter 3

Failure to deliver: ethical issues relating to epidural analgesia in uncomplicated labour

Rosemary Mander

INTRODUCTION: AN HISTORICAL ANALOGY

The outstanding event in the history of pain relief in childbirth was the first administration of ether for a delivery by Doctor (later Sir) James Young Simpson in Edinburgh in January 1847. (Moir 1973 p 1)

While not underestimating Simpson's achievement in overcoming the opposition of an entrenched medical establishment to the alleviation of women's pain in labour, the introduction of this form of pain control was not totally devoid of damaging side-effects. This is apparent from contemporaneous accounts of the use of chloroform analgesia, which was introduced later in the same year. These side-effects include a reduction in uterine activity, which was associated with prolonged labour, as well as other, more life-threatening hazards (Smith 1979). These adverse side-effects clearly did not manifest themselves in the postprandial research undertaken at the Simpson dinner table. Despite this, chloroform analgesia was generally accepted, to the extent that by 13 years later it was 'almost universally employed' (Smith 1979 p 22).

The introduction of epidural analgesia into the birthing room just over a century later (Morris 2001) has certain features in common with the advent of ether and chloroform. These similarities go far beyond the intended effect of pain control; they even go beyond the pharmacological side-effect of weakening uterine contractions. Both of these innovations have contributed to the transfer of control over the birth from the mother to her medical attendant. Both innovations involve a perceived ideal solution by medical practitioners to the problem of pain in labour. Each of these innovations carried with it certain advantages for both mother and obstetrician; each also carried a plethora of side-effects which for the mother would have been hazards, had they not also presented obstetricians with both reason and opportunity to extend and utilise their rapidly developing interventive skills. Similarly, epidural analgesia comprised a technique that offered for the obstetric anaesthetist, an entrée to the birthing room and a route to achieve recognition and professional status (Mander 1993b).

The use of epidural analgesia in uncomplicated labour, like the less well-documented effects of ether and chloroform, raises a number of issues, many of them carrying serious ethical implications. As already mentioned, when such forms of pain control are used, the woman's control over her birth experience is markedly reduced; this has been described in pathophysiological terms (Jouppila et al 1980, Williams et al 1985) and is recognised as an example of the 'cascade of intervention' (Varney Burst 1983). Chloroform analgesia was associated with a reduction in uterine activity and this, together with greater feasibility, increased the incidence of instrumental intervention for the birth (Tew 1995). In the context of epidural analgesia, the cascade of intervention involves the weakening of uterine contractions as well as certain neurological changes that decrease the tone of the pelvic floor, leading to incomplete rotation of the presenting part; that is, the fetal head in uncomplicated labour (Morris 2001). Oxytocic drugs, utilised to overcome the associated delay in labour, increase the risk of fetal hypoxia and the need for instrumental or even surgical intervention for the birth (Evans 1992, Keirse & Chalmers 1989). The link between epidural analgesia and surgical birth (caesarean) remains contentious. Ramin et al (1995) found in their randomised controlled trial (RCT) that a two- to fourfold increased risk of caesarean birth is associated with epidural analgesia in both nulliparous and parous women. Loughnan et al (2000), however, found in a UK RCT that this link is not supported. Such conflicting findings may not be surprising in view of the obvious impossibility of blinding attendants to the group to which the women have been randomised.

In attempting to overcome at least some of the problems of epidural analgesia, the low dose or mobile technique has been introduced (Morris 2001). The Comparative Obstetric Mobile Epidural Trial (COMET 2001) has shown that the proportion of spontaneous vaginal births may be increased by using this technique, but only to about 43% of births. In this study the number of births assisted by instruments was reduced. The cost of these improved maternal outcomes seems to be in the poorer condition of the neonate, whose APGAR scores were lower and who was more likely to need active resuscitation.

AUTONOMY

The reduction in or loss of bodily control over her labour may also apply at a higher, more intellectual level in that the mother's control over her personal decision-making, that is her autonomy, may equally be under threat. The challenge to the mother's autonomy derives from the series of events or 'cascade' that may follow the administration of epidural analgesia.

In a childbearing situation, the various participants may be regarded, or regard themselves, as requiring some degree of autonomy. The balance of autonomy has been observed to be changing for our medical colleagues since the consumerist approach has become a threat to their self-determination (Pellegrino 1994). Similarly, in association with certain governmental initiatives (Department of Health 1993, House of Commons 1992), the midwife may find it necessary to negotiate a *modus vivendi* with the mother to ensure that both retain a mutually acceptable degree of autonomy (Mander 1993a). The mother's autonomy has recently assumed greater significance due to cultural developments, such as consumerism and the women's movement, and due to organisational changes within the UK health care system, such as the Patients' Charter. The ability of health care systems such as the UK National Health Service (NHS) to meet the mother's need for autonomy and to provide 'choice in childbirth' has long been questioned (Mander 1993c, Richards 1982).

In health care situations, such as childbearing, the priority that we attach to autonomy leads us to apply it in the form of the ethical principle of respect for autonomy. Such respect manifests itself in our encouragement of autonomous decision-making by clients and patients, an essential feature of which, clearly founded on and arising out of respect for autonomy, is consent to treatment.

SUBLIMINAL EFFECTS

In considering the elements that create an environment in which 'autonomous authorisation' is feasible, Beauchamp & Childress (1994) begin by dismissing competence as a threshold requirement on largely practical grounds. The other two salient components of consent are voluntariness and information. It is necessary for us to consider how these two elements may be threatened in the context of epidural analgesia in uncomplicated labour.

The concept of coercion becomes relevant in the present context by the 'credible or severe threat of harm or force to [exert] control another' (Beauchamp & Childress 1994 p 164). These credible or severe threats need not be externally applied. The labour pains that a mother experiences may lead her to anticipate 'harm' in the form of yet more unbearable pain if she declines the analgesic method that may be being dangled tantalisingly in front of her.

Only marginally less subtle is the way in which midwives and other relatively intimate carers may influence the mother's decision-making in labour. This influence may exert its effect in any number of different ways, but possibly by slanting the way in which the available choices are presented. This effective limitation of the mother's decision-making may be regarded as quite a subtle form of coercion. Evidence to support this suggestion is currently merely anecdotal, having been observed by chance during a large and authoritative study of mothers' experience of epidural analgesia (Perry, personal communication). Mothers being cared for by certain individual midwives were found to be consistently either more or less likely to choose epidural analgesia. It may be that this anecdotal observation may derive from other factors unrelated to the midwife's personality, attitudes or behaviour. The phenomenon observed by Perry may, alternatively, have been associated with the mother's chance perception of benefits. Further alternative explanations are that certain midwives may have been systematically allocated to care for more 'epidural-prone' mothers, or that some midwives may be less well able to cope with the mother's pain or with her way of articulating her pain. It is not possible to assess which of these underlying factors applies without the collection of further data. Perry's observation of the carer's contribution, though, is supported by our knowledge of the limited objectivity in their administration of analgesic agents. These decisions have been clearly shown to be subjective and vulnerable to stereotyping (McDonald 1994).

Such influence, pressure or coercion by nursing/midwifery staff has, however, been clearly demonstrated in the context of a different intervention in childbearing. The objectivity of clinical decision-making in relation to caesareans has been called into question (Enkin 1989). Against this background Radin et al (1993) used a retrospective research design to study the caesarean rates among 31 labour ward nurses in a North American hospital.

The nurses were categorised according to the caesarean rates among their healthy, nulliparous 'patients' in spontaneous labour. These researchers found a consistent variation between the nurses in the proportion of 'low-risk' mothers in their care who gave birth by caesarean. The caesarean rates of the individual nurses varied between 4.9% and 19% of the mothers for whom each nurse cared. These differences could not be accounted for in the age, parity, socio-economic status, physician in attendance, epidural use, acceleration of labour, stage of labour, baby's weight or gestational age.

The patients of those nurses least associated with caesarean were also less likely to have a long labour or a vaginal birth assisted by instruments. The lower rates of interventive birth were found not to be associated with any fetal/neonatal ill-effects. The researchers do, however, link these outcomes with the increased likelihood of the nurses with low caesarean rates obtaining and utilising psychosocial data about the mothers in their care. This suggests that these nurses took a more woman-oriented approach to care, which may have reinforced the mother's confidence and enabled her to labour physiologically. Contrary to my earlier suggestion that certain midwives may be systematically allocated to care for certain 'types' of mothers, Radin and her colleagues could find no consistent organisational factor that would explain the difference between the nurses' caesarean rates.

Similarly, more direct associations between individual midwives and high or low intervention rates are well-established. A study of midwives' episiotomy rates clearly showed the association between an individual midwife's care and the likelihood of the mother sustaining this form of deliberate perineal damage (Wilkerson 1984). She reviewed the birth records of 2933 mothers who were cared for at the birth in one unit by 21 midwives during a 12-month period. This figure constitutes 56.4% of the births in the maternity unit concerned; the remaining births were medically supervised. Each midwife was identified by a letter of the alphabet, in order of their frequency of performing an episiotomy. The chances of the mother sustaining an episiotomy varied hugely. A mother being cared for by midwife A was over ten times more likely to encounter this form of perineal damage than her sister who was being cared for by midwife U. Of the primigravidae cared for by midwife A, 92.8% sustained an episiotomy, whereas only 3% of multigravidae cared for by midwife U sustained one.

While the huge variation in midwives' practice is apparent from Wilkerson's data, it is necessary to question why midwives like midwife A practised in such a 'scissor-happy', though far from unique, manner (Inch 1982). Protecting the integrity of the pelvic floor and the fetal brain have been cited as the rationale for episiotomy, but changing attitudes may have been more significant. Attitudes are likely to have been influenced by midwives' own statutory bodies, the (then) Central Midwives Boards, who in 1967 incorporated perineal infiltration and episiotomy into midwifery training. A further influence was the surgical orientation of midwives' medical colleagues (Wilkerson 1984), which increased the pressure on midwives to intervene in this way. This pressure carried serious implications for mothers' autonomy and midwives' decision-making as evidenced by the emergence of the 'routine prophylactic episiotomy' (Formato, 1985).

Episiotomy is clearly a particularly direct example of midwives' influence over interventions. It is necessary to consider the possibility of more subtle pressure such as in the use of episiotomy. The more subtle effects have been shown in both the research-based observations relating to caesarean and the more anecdotal evidence concerning epidural analgesia, mentioned earlier.

MIDWIVES' INSIDER KNOWLEDGE

As well as the voluntariness of the mother's decision being influenced more or less subliminally by the midwife's attitudes and information-giving, the decision may also be influenced by the midwife's specialist knowledge. The mother's decision to accept or not accept an offer of epidural analgesia may be affected by the midwife's knowledge of the person who will be siting (inserting into the epidural space) the epidural cannula and local anaesthetic. The midwife may be aware of the level of technical skills of the obstetric anaesthetist on call. Even obstetric anaesthetists admit the existence of and dangers associated with the practice of unskilled anaesthetists (Morgan 1987), so it is hardly surprising that midwives may come to question the standard of the technical expertise of some of their anaesthetic colleagues. Clearly, a midwife's ability to encourage a mother to accept epidural analgesia is likely to be influenced by the midwife's assessment, based on previous observational experience, of the expertise of the practitioner who is on call at the relevant time. In the same way as midwives may seek to protect the mothers in their care from an unskilled anaesthetist, they may similarly seek to protect them from a less than satisfactory interpersonal encounter. While the siting of an epidural cannula may not be an intensely painful procedure, it is not always easy for a mother in labour to remain still and in a suitable position. As one mother told Oakley (1993), 'I found it very hard to keep still on my side in labour with needles being put in my back. Especially when a pain came' (p 104).

A certain amount of coaxing and encouragement may be necessary from the anaesthetist. While the communication skills of the obstetric anaesthetist may make this arduous procedure easier and less tiresome, some anaesthetists may lack the high level of interpersonal skills to achieve this. The midwife may judge that the likelihood of a disturbing interpersonal encounter for the mother may not be justified in view of the level of pain the mother is perceived to be facing and, thus, discourage her implicitly or openly from choosing epidural analgesia. Thus the midwife's knowledge of the personnel likely to be involved may influence the voluntariness of the mother's epidural decision.

PRESSURE OF BIAS

Draper (see Chapter 1) links coercion with the way in which information is presented to the client or patient. Draper's examples include, first, the order in which the various options are recounted to the mother; although she does not indicate whether those higher on the list are more likely to be favoured or vice versa. Second, Draper explains how pressure may be applied by unduly emphasising either the benefits of a certain, favoured, course of action or the hazards or damaging side-effects of the less favourable course of action. Information given to the mother relating to epidural analgesia may employ both of these strategies; an example of the latter use of emphasis is found in an informational booklet distributed to all mothers in one NHS Trust: 'Epidurals do not cause sleepiness in the baby in the same way as an injection of diamorphine or pethidine' (Stewart & West undated).

By way of support for Draper's comments, the use of the hard sell to persuade the mother to accept epidural analgesia has been observed and reported by campaigning organisations. Some of these organisations attempt to preserve the mother's control over her birth experience by ensuring the voluntariness of her decision-making (Robinson 1993).

EXPECTATION OF FAILURE

As in many situations in life and in some relating to childbearing, women learn of the risk of failure at an early stage. The mother's voluntary decision-making may be limited by pressure deriving from the expectation of failure. If this expectation is held, however unconsciously, by those near her, it may undermine the confidence of the mother. As Tew (1995) observes, confidence is fundamentally important to successful, physiological childbearing. She suggests that obstetricians have sought to establish their professional status by winning public confidence through 'destroying the confidence of mothers in their own reproductive efficiency' (1995 p 11, 133). Tew observes that the confidence of other carers, such as midwives, was also destroyed. This undermining of women's self-confidence began with the introduction of antenatal care in the early years of the 20th century (Tew 1995). A similar strategy was employed to persuade mothers and midwives of the 'total safety' of hospital birth (Beech 1992 p 155).

Particularly vulnerable is the mother's confidence in her own ability to labour successfully and physiologically. The expectation of failure to cope with the physiological processes of labour is shared by staff as well as mothers and has resulted in the hard sell mentioned (Robinson 1993). Another example of the expectation of failure is the traditional education about breastfeeding, which features details of the associated problems, such as breast engorgement, cracked nipples, inadequate milk supply and mastitis (Blumfield 1992). Such 'education' tends to be provided alongside details of formula feeding (Watson & Mander 1995). In this way, the mother's confidence in her ability to breastfeed is undermined, while a less healthy message is transmitted through supposedly health promotional material. The expectation of failure may be held by a variety of formal and informal carers with whom the mother is in contact prior to and during her labour. These carers or agents can be divided, for convenience, into four groups: the formal carers, the informal carers, policy makers and other mothers.

The formal carers: midwives and medical staff

Differing expectations became apparent in a research project undertaken by Walker (1972, 1976), which distinguished the approaches of midwives and their medical colleagues. The midwives were clearly able to assume a waiting role during labour, in the expectation that, given time, nature would effectively take its course and result in a healthy outcome. The medical staff, on the other hand, regarded every labour as potentially pathological until it was safely completed, thus requiring their personal supervision, availability and enthusiasm for intervention at all times. The medical expectation of failure in childbearing has been summarised by Percival (1970) in his oft-quoted aphorism 'labour is only normal in retrospect'.

It may be that, because obstetricians during their training are unlikely to observe more than a small number of normal labours and in the course of their practice none at all, they have difficulty anticipating a physiological outcome to labour. In the same way, obstetric anaesthetists tend not to be involved with a mother who is coping well with her pain in labour, and thus may have difficulty envisaging the prospect of an unmedicated labour. In addition to their other reasons for advocating the increasing use of epidural analgesia in uncomplicated labour (Mander 1993b), limited experience of women coping may engender in obstetric anaesthetists the expectation of failure to cope.

Informal and cultural influences

While clearly apparent in some situations, the expectation of failure to cope with pain in labour may not operate in certain other cultures. One such culture, which has been the focus of considerable interest and some research attention, is the Netherlands. It is generally assumed that the Dutch mother's ability to cope with labour pain unassisted by medication is learned behaviour that may be culturally determined. As Tasharrofi (1993) observes, the result is that analgesia is 'neither expected nor required'. The important cultural component in the acceptance or otherwise of labour pain has been attributed to some cultures' adherence to the medical model of health (van Teijlingen 1994).

To illustrate this differing orientation, Senden and colleagues (1988) undertook a study comparing the expectations and experiences of labour pain in mothers in Iowa (USA) and Nijmegen (Netherlands). In a sample of 256, a large majority of Dutch mothers

(79.2%) did not use medication to control labour pain whereas this applied to only 37.6% of American mothers. The proportions in each group showing satisfaction with their method of pain control and the fulfilment of their expectations of pain showed no significant differences. These authors consider that their findings reflect attitudes which are derived from the confidence of Dutch women, learned through personal, family and social experience, in their own ability to cope with labour pain and to labour successfully.

Policy factors

A further factor, not unrelated to the previous two, which may be involved in the way in which the mother's expectation of failure may limit the voluntariness of her decision-making, is the organisational aspects of her childbearing experience as determined by local and national health policy. By this I mean the location of childbirth for the vast majority of mothers in the UK; that is, in a hospital. Inevitably and probably correctly, hospitalisation carries with it an aura of illness, which is transposed to the physiological process of childbearing. Thus birth is transformed into a potentially pathological process and in need of safety precautions, possibly in the form of medical interventions, to prevent dire consequences. Macfarlane (1992) maintains that the safety argument is founded on the observation that mortality rates are currently lower than they were when home birth was more easily available and happened more generally. As a result, she argues, hospital birth is assumed to be the *cause* of lower mortality rates. In this way the notion of safety is used to justify the currently high hospital birth rates and to intimidate women into giving birth in hospital (Beech 1991). Hence, organisational factors raise the expectation of failure in the mother and further limit the voluntariness of her decision-making.

Other mothers' 'old wives' tales'

Personal observation leads me to believe that mothers themselves may, probably inadvertently, encourage in each other the expectation of failure. This is through the phenomena that have been referred to as 'old wives' tales' and 'new wives' tales' (Perkins 1980). These are the traditional, as well as more modern, horror stories that mothers have since time immemorial shared with mothers-to-be. My own observation indicates that 'old wives' tales' not infrequently focus on labour pain. This focus emphasises the severity, the duration and the irremediable nature of this pain. These stories clearly serve to help the telling mother to adjust to her experience of childbirth and may help her to restore her self-esteem after what she may perceive to have been a disappointing experience. The benefits, however, for the mother-to-be are less obvious and may serve to arouse in her the expectation of failure to cope.

Taking a broader view, we see that the expectation of failure features prominently in the folklore of childbirth. While the prospect of maternal death has thankfully receded, the spectres of other failures have assumed greater significance. These spectres have been used to advantage by certain groups to achieve ends that are not solely for the benefit of the mother and her baby. The speciality of obstetric anaesthesia was initially introduced to solve the problem of an intransigent maternal death rate. It has, however, developed into a profession by fostering in mothers the expectation of their inability to cope with the pain of uncomplicated labour and by offering an intervention to prevent that pain (Mander 1993b, 1994). Through the modification of mothers' expectations and the development and maintenance of a professional group, on both an individual and a cultural basis, the widespread use of epidural analgesia has served to limit the voluntary decision-making or autonomy of childbearing women.

INFORMATION

The demarcation between obtaining consent and giving adequate information is not always easily distinguishable. This is because consent, unless preceded by giving the patient or client relevant information, is worthless. Lindley (1991) spells out the possible repercussions for the practitioner in terms of, first, being guilty of battery and second, rendering the practitioner open to claims for damages. He maintains that such claims would be likely to be upheld regardless of whether the patient was injured, whether the practitioner was negligent or whether consent would have been forthcoming had it been sought.

The standard of information-giving may be measured according to the professional practice standard, the reasonable person standard or the subjective standard (Beauchamp & Childress 1994, Henderson 1994).

QUALITY OF THE INFORMATION RELATING TO EPIDURAL ANALGESIA

The quantity of the information that is given to the patient or client varies according to which of these standards is operating. The quality of that information may also vary according to an even broader range of determinants. This may be seen to apply in the context of epidural analgesia in uncomplicated labour. The quality of the information may be affected by exogenous factors, such as the existence or non-existence of relevant research, or may be biased by endogenous factors such as personal and professional attitudes.

The research basis

As in so many aspects of maternity care, the research evidence on which our practice is based is far from sufficient to allow the mother to give fully informed consent to her care (Chalmers 1993). The lack of authoritative research evidence places the midwife and, more importantly, the mother in a quandary about the most appropriate care for mother and baby. Richards (1982) observes that, like many interventions in childbearing, epidural analgesia was introduced for the benefit of a small number of women to avoid serious, that is of life threatening, problems. On the basis of positive experiences for these few women, and without the benefit of randomised controlled trials of its efficacy, this form of pain control was made available to large numbers of mothers experiencing uncomplicated childbirth (Chalmers 1993). This medical logic was summarised succinctly by Baird et al (1953 p 27) when they said: 'If it is accepted that [this intervention] is safer for certain types of patient where the risks are high, it must also be safer where the risks are less.' Like research into the benefits and hazards of other frequently used interventions in childbearing, such as ultrasound, after approximately 40 years of widespread use it is becoming too late to put the genie back into the bottle. The research that was neglected when these techniques were in their infancy may no longer be feasible.

The research evidence that is available is limited in its scope, being largely confined to the technical aspects of epidural analgesia, and not well utilised in practice. This is apparent in a booklet for mothers that, while promoting the epidural, fails to mention practically the only research evidence on this topic about which there is confidence (Howell & Chalmers 1992). The increased use of instruments to assist the birth is omitted, with barely passing but reassuring reference to second-stage delay: 'During the second stage of labour the urge to, "bear down," may be reduced, but your midwife is trained to help you bear down when it is appropriate' (Stewart & West undated).

The conspiracy of, if not silence at least misinformation, is perpetuated in a leaflet for mothers published by the Obstetric

Anaesthetists Association (OAA undated). This assures the mother '[y]ou are more likely to have a normal delivery than any other type of delivery' (p 8). Such a careful choice of words would clearly be reassuring for anyone seeking reassurance. Accurate information, however, is absent. The general lack of relevant research-based information is apparent in a number of crucial areas relating to epidural analgesia in uncomplicated labour.

Long-term effects

Partly because the mother's stay in the maternity unit is becoming shorter and partly because her care lacks continuity, the long-term effects of epidural analgesia in labour have passed largely unnoticed. Kitzinger's (1987) methodologically odd study was the first to draw our attention to the neurological and orthopaedic sequelae of epidural analgesia in uncomplicated labour (Mander 1994). Although large ($n = 908$), Kitzinger's sample comprised National Childbirth Trust volunteers in the UK and Australia. The sample was self-selected, uncontrolled and, presumably, highly motivated. There were approximately equal numbers from each country. Drawing on the experiences of this sample in a qualitative research design, Kitzinger reports an epidural failure rate of 15%, as well as more serious problems such as sudden hypotensive episodes and dural tap. Kitzinger mentions that 18% of the sample perceived themselves to be suffering from long-term side-effects including neurological and orthopaedic symptoms. The emotional sequelae, such as regrets and feelings of failure, were found to be delayed for weeks, months or even until the birth of the next baby.

While Kitzinger's research project may obviously be criticised for the selection of the sample, the researcher makes no unjustified claims about whether her conclusions can be generalised. She does not use the term, but her work indicates the existence of the 'cascade of intervention' in the experiences of her informants. The reception accorded to the far more authoritative study by MacArthur et al (1992) was barely more accepting of the incapacitating and enduring effects of this form of pain control. Despite the findings of MacArthur et al being initially disregarded for sampling reasons and their veracity being denied, they have been accepted, albeit reluctantly (Robinson 1993).

MacArthur's original aim (1991) was to study the long-term health implications of pregnancy and childbearing. This retrospective study was large and the sampling and methodological detail is comprehensive. The data illuminate the wide-ranging, pervasive and enduring health problems following childbirth. The data on the long-term health sequelae associated with the use of epidural analgesia in labour are consistent with Kitzinger's (1987) findings. MacArthur and her colleagues (1992) found that 19.3% of mothers who gave birth vaginally while using epidural analgesia developed long-term backache, whereas only 10.4% of those mothers who gave birth vaginally without epidural analgesia did so. For some mothers who had used epidural analgesia, the backache was accompanied by headache, migraine, shoulder/neckaches, pain/weakness of limbs or tingling of the extremities.

The hypothesis advanced by MacArthur is that these neurological and orthopaedic sequelae are associated with subclinical trauma to the spinal axis during labour. She maintains that the minor discomforts that ordinarily cause a person to adjust their posture are neither perceptible nor correctable under the effect of epidural analgesia. These traumas later manifest themselves as symptoms due to the superimposed stress of caring for a young baby.

This debate was joined by MacLeod et al (1995), who contributed data collected prior to the media attention attracted by MacArthur's work. These obstetric anaesthetists surveyed 2065 mothers one year after the birth and achieved a 67.1% response rate. Of the mothers who had used epidural analgesia, 26.2% were found to have developed new long-term backache since the birth. Of those mothers not exposed to epidural analgesia, only 1.7% developed backache.

The use to which these research findings have been put may not accord with the intentions of the researchers. This may mean, as Robinson observes, informing a mother who is not coping with her labour pain that '[a]n epidural could cause you long term backache—do you still want it?' (Robinson 1993 p 28). This may not be the most appropriate use of this information. Obstetric anaesthetists have worked hard in an effort to overcome this adverse publicity. Their defence relies heavily on claims that women had forgotten that their back pain preceded the administration of the epidural (Reynolds & Russell 1998). This argument is condescendingly unconvincing.

Mother–oriented concerns

The limited research attention focused on the concerns of mothers relating to pain control methods compares dismally with the generous research attention given to issues relating to the technique of administering epidural analgesia (Mander 1994). It is necessary to question whether this focus reflects the medical view of research in more general terms. The 'scientific' approach espoused by our medical colleagues values the measurement of phenomena, such as physiological observations. Such measurements carry the reassuring certainty that they are incontrovertible and, thus, valuable. The reverse may equally apply, to the extent that phenomena that are not measurable may be denied, disregarded or dismissed as of no value. For these reasons mothers' responses to pain control have been given only superficial research attention, and have sought largely to persuade the active birth movement of the errors of its ways (Mander 1994).

Researchers who have undertaken authoritative studies into the mother's feelings and expectations during childbearing indicate that perceptions of being in control are crucial to the mother's satisfaction with her experience (Green et al 1990). The effects of the method of pain control on the mother's perception of control also require research attention; this would enable carers to give to the mother who wishes to retain control during childbirth the information that would allow her to do so (Mander 1992). Oakley (1993), in her follow-up to a major research project does, however, identify how much the effectiveness of epidural analgesia is appreciated by mothers. She endorses Green et al's findings, though, by observing that mothers are far less satisfied with their feelings of diminished control, together with other side-effects and long-term health problems. In her conclusion Oakley reports the integrated view that mothers adopt of their birth experience, including the pain. She regrets that researchers are less able to reflect this holistic view of birth, tending to make measurements and ask simplistic questions about satisfaction. The researcher's distinction between physical and emotional phenomena does not appear to match the mother's experience. Oakley argues that the orientation of research needs to be adapted in order to combine emotional as well as physical aspects of pain. In this way it may become possible to provide the mother with the information that she needs before consenting to an intervention such as epidural analgesia.

Failure rates

Local and personal success rates are an example of the information with physical and emotional implications that needs to be made available to mothers, prior to valid decisions being made about pain control in labour. This aspect of epidural analgesia is not considered serious enough to warrant publication, even less research attention (Crawford 1986), and a light-hearted chapter entitled 'They think it's all over', reflects this attitude (Reynolds 1997). Writing about non-pharmacological methods of pain control, Simkin (1989) briefly indicates the success rates of lumbar epidural analgesia as being between 67% and 90%. Additionally, one of the few studies to even mention the possibility of epidural failure is the much-criticised work by Kitzinger (1987), which reports an epidural failure rate of 15%.

The reason for my plea for more research-based information on this topic lies in the serious implications of a failed epidural for the mother and for her carers. In this situation the mother is likely to have prepared herself for a little discomfort, but certainly not for the full-blown experience of labour pain. Despite the best efforts of our anaesthetic colleagues the problem may not be resolved. Not surprisingly I have found mothers in this situation to be disappointed and angry as well as suffering pain for which they had not prepared themselves either physically or emotionally. As a midwife I have had to draw on my full repertoire of caring and interpersonal skills to support mothers through this doubly negative experience.

The difficulty that our anaesthetic colleagues encounter in facing the possibility of a failed epidural was impressed on me on one such occasion. The most senior anaesthetist had been summoned to resolve the apparently intractable problem of an unsupported mother's failed epidural. In response to this dismal scenario, she asked the miserable, frightened and angry young woman 'Why are you making all this fuss? I had four without an epidural and I never made all this noise.'

Professional factors

As well as factors relating to the existence of appropriate information about epidural analgesia, we need to consider how and whether such information as exists is transmitted to the mother for her use. Inevitably, the information in this context is largely unidirectional; that is, from the practitioner to the mother. Paternalism, which has been mentioned already, may operate alone or, in certain situations, may become entangled with professional relationships to affect information-giving. These relationships may be interprofessional, interoccupational or client–professional. Regardless of the personnel involved, there are serious implications for the transmission of information and, eventually, decision-making.

Interoccupational relationships have been shown by Kirkham (1989) to influence adversely information given by personnel and occupational groups perceived as being of different status. Kirkham's finding was that, in the presence of colleagues perceived to be of higher status, carers were less likely to inform the labouring mother of choices and developments. Because the higher-status staff did not consider such information-giving as part of their remit, the mother found herself even less well informed after the arrival of the 'expert'.

Meredith (1993) researched the implications of medical dominance for the operation of consent in a general surgical setting. Because of their poor impressions of the intellectual abilities of their patients 'the surgeons ... were not enthusiastic at the prospect of devoting more time to discussing surgical alternatives, risks and complications, and outlook indicators for their patients' benefit'. It may be that, in childbearing, medical dominance is less oppressive due to the absence of illness. The contribution of illness, however, is probably small, if it exists, but of far greater significance is the part played by power relationships. Freidson (1970) suggests that even though terms such as 'professional' have become devalued by wider educational opportunities, their underlying feature remains unchanged and this feature is power. In this context power relates to the ability to control one's work through education and legislation as well as on a more mundane basis, by controlling the market within which one operates. Despite the reforms in the UK health care system it is clear that power, as defined by Freidson, has been retained by our medical colleagues to a far greater extent than by other health care providers or by health care consumers. Freidson questions whether in future this power may be worth less, due to the increasing specialisation of industries, which may include health care. He optimistically considers that increasing fragmentation of the professions will give rise to a need for cooperation between the different occupational groups and, inevitably, the consumer. If Freidson is right, the mother's input into decision-making is likely to increase.

CONCLUSION

I have questioned the ethical basis on which epidural services are provided for the mother experiencing uncomplicated labour. Certain organisational and occupational factors have been shown to reduce the likelihood of the mother being able to give valid consent. The lack of appropriate research-based information and the limited preparedness of those involved to communicate the relevant information that does exist further reduce this likelihood.

Throughout this chapter the possibility of failure has featured prominently. The acceptance of epidural services has been fostered by the expectation that mothers will fail to cope with the pain of uncomplicated labour.

The development of epidural services has not been supported by research into those areas of pain control that are likely to be of concern to mothers, such as success rates, long-term side-effects and non-life-threatening side-effects. Thus the mother's need for information cannot be sufficiently satisfied to enable her to decide on and give valid consent to the most appropriate form of pain control. Significant among the information on epidural analgesia that has not been provided is the failure rate of this intervention.

While decisions about the introduction of innovative methods of pain control for use in labour may, in the past, have been made in fashionable Edinburgh dining rooms, such innovation is no longer acceptable. Before the mother is able to give her proper and fully informed consent to interventions such as epidural analgesia, certain requirements need to be satisfied. The first is that the mother is confident that there is no reason why she should not be physiologically, psychologically and emotionally able to cope with the pain of uncomplicated labour. The second is that she is aware of the implications of such interventions, for herself in the short and long term, for her labour, and for her baby. This information must include the possibility of the intervention failing to meet her expectations.

References

Baird D, Thomson A, Duncan E 1953 The causes and prevention of stillbirths and first week deaths; part II: evidence from Aberdeen clinical records. Journal of Obstetrics and Gynaecology of the British Empire 60:17–30

Beauchamp T L, Childress J F 1994 Principles of biomedical ethics, 4th edn. Oxford University Press, Oxford

Beech B L 1991 Home birth: what kind of choice? AIMS Quarterly Journal 3:6–7, 20

Beech B L 1992 Women's views of childbirth. In: Chard T & Richards M P M (eds) Obstetrics in the 1990s: current controversies. MacKeith Press, London

Blumfield W 1992 Life after birth: every woman's guide to the first year of motherhood. Element Books, Shaftesbury, Dorset

Chalmers I 1993 Effective care in midwifery: research, the professions and the public. Midwives Chronicle 106:3–12

Comparative Obstetric Mobile Epidural Trial Study Group UK (COMET) 2001
Effect of low-dose mobile versus traditional epidural techniques on mode of
delivery: a randomised controlled trial. Lancet 358:19–23

Crawford J S 1986 Some maternal complications of epidural analgesia for labour.
Obstetric Anaesthesia Digest 6: 221–222

Department of Health 1993 Changing childbirth: report of the expert maternity
group. HMSO, London

Enkin M 1989 Commentary: why do the caesarean section rates differ? Birth 16:
207–208

Evans S 1992 The value of cardiotocograph monitoring in midwifery. Midwives
Chronicle 105:4–11

Formato L S 1985 Routine prophylactic episiotomy. Journal of Nurse-Midwifery 30:3

Freidson E 1970 Profession of medicine. Mead & Co, New York

Green J M, Coupland V A, Kitzinger J V 1990 Expectations, experiences and
psychological outcomes of childbirth: a prospective study of 825 women. Birth
17:15–24

Henderson M 1994 Risk and the doctor–patient relationship. In: Gillon R,
Lloyd A (eds) Principles of health care ethics. John Wiley, Chichester, p 435–444

House of Commons 1992 Health committee second report, maternity services.
HMSO, London

Howell C J, Chalmers I 1992 A review of prospectively controlled comparisons of
epidural with non-epidural forms of pain relief during labour. International
Journal of Obstetric Anaesthesia 1:93–110

Inch S 1982 Birthrights. Hutchinson, London

Jouppila R et al 1980 The effect of segmental epidural analgesia on maternal
prolactin during labour. British Journal of Obstetrics and Gynaecology
31:234–238

Keirse M J N C, Chalmers I 1989 Methods for inducing labour. In: Chalmers I,
Enkin M, Keirse M J N C (eds) Effective care in pregnancy and childbirth
volume 2: childbirth. Oxford University Press, Oxford, p 1507–1579

Kirkham M 1989 Midwives and information-giving during labour. In:
Robinson S, Thomson A M (eds) Midwives, research and childbirth volume 1.
Chapman & Hall, London, p 117–138

Kitzinger S 1987 Some women's experiences of epidurals—a descriptive study.
National Childbirth Trust, London

Lindley R 1991 Informed consent and the ghost of Bolam. In: Brazier M,
Lobjoit M (eds) Protecting the vulnerable: autonomy and consent in health
care. Routledge, London, p 134–149

Loughnan B A et al 2000 Randomised controlled comparison of epidural
bupivacaine versus pethidine for analgesia in labour. British Journal of
Anaesthesia 84:715–719

MacArthur C 1991 Health after childbirth. HMSO, London

MacArthur C, Lewis M, Knox E G 1992 Investigation of long-term problems after
obstetric epidural anaesthesia. British Medical Journal 304:1279–1282

McDonald D D 1994 Gender and ethnic stereotyping and narcotic analgesic
administration. Research in Nursing and Health 17:45–49

Macfarlane A 1992 Interpreting statistics. Nursing Times 88:62

MacLeod J et al 1995 Backache and epidural analgesia. International Journal of
Obstetric Anaesthesia 4:21–25

Mander R 1992 The control of pain in labour. Journal of Clinical Nursing 1:219–223

Mander R 1993a Autonomy in midwifery and maternity care. Midwives
    Chronicle 106:369–374
Mander R 1993b Epidural analgesia 1: recent history. British Journal of Midwifery
    2:259–264
Mander R 1993c Who chooses the choices? Modern Midwife 3:23–25
Mander R 1994 Epidural analgesia: 2. Research basis. British Journal of Midwifery
    2:12–16
Meredith P 1993 Patient participation in decision-making and consent to treatment:
    the case of general surgery. Sociology of Health and Illness 15:315–336
Moir D D 1973 Pain relief in labour: a handbook for midwives, 2nd edn. Churchill
    Livingstone, Edinburgh
Morgan B M 1987 Mortality and anaesthesia. In: Morgan B M (ed) Foundations of
    obstetric anaesthesia. Farrand Press, London, p 255–270
Morris P J 2001 Epidural analgesia: historical summary and present practice.
    British Journal of Midwifery 9:36–40
Oakley A 1993 The follow-up survey. In: Chamberlain G, Wraigh T A, Steer P
    (eds) Pain and its relief in childbirth. Churchill Livingstone, Edinburgh
Obstetric Anaesthetists Association (OAA) Undated Pain relief in labour.
    Obstetric Anaesthetists Association, London
Pellegrino E D 1994 The four principles and the doctor–patient relationship: the
    need for a better linkage. In: Gillon R, Lloyd A (eds) Principles of health care
    ethics. John Wiley, Chichester, p 353–366
Percival R C 1970 Management of normal labour. The Practitioner 204:1221–1224
Perkins E R 1980 Education for childbirth and parenthood. Croom Helm, London
Radin T G, Harmon J S, Hanson D A 1993 Nurses' care during labor: its effect on
    the cesarean birth rate of healthy, nulliparous women. Birth 20:14–21
Ramin S et al 1995 Randomised trial of epidural versus intravenous analgesia
    during labour. Obstetrics and Gynecology 86:783–789
Reynolds F 1997 They think it's all over. In: Russell R, Scrutton M, Porter J (eds)
    Pain relief in labour. BMJ Publishing Group, London, p 220–242
Reynolds F, Russell R 1998 Epidural anaesthesia does not cause long term
    backache. British Medical Journal 316:69–70
Richards M P M 1982 The trouble with 'choice' in childbirth. Birth 9:253–260
Robinson J 1993 Long term consequence of epidurals and other childbirth care.
    AIMS Quarterly Journal 5:27–28
Senden I P M et al 1988 Labour pain: a comparison of parturients in a Dutch and
    an American teaching hospital. Obstetrics & Gynecology 71:451–453
Simkin P 1989 Non-pharmacological methods of pain control. In: Chalmers I,
    Enkin M, Keirse M J N C (eds) Effective care in pregnancy and childbirth 2.
    Oxford University Press, Oxford, p 893–912
Smith FB 1979 The people's health 1830–1910. Holmes & Meier, New York
Stewart M, West C Undated The birth of your baby at the Simpson. Royal
    Infirmary Trust, Edinburgh
Tasharrofi A 1993 Midwifery care in the Netherlands. Midwives Chronicle
    106:286–288
Tew M 1995 Safer childbirth? A critical history of maternity care. Chapman &
    Hall, London
van Teijlingen E 1994 A social or medical model of childbirth? Comparing the
    arguments in Grampian (Scotland) and the Netherlands. Unpublished PhD
    thesis, University of Aberdeen

Varney Burst H 1983 The influence of consumers in the birthing movement. Topics in Clinical Nursing 5:42–54

Walker J 1972 The changing role of the midwife. International Journal of Nursing Studies 9:85–94

Walker J 1976 Midwife or obstetric nurse? Some perceptions of midwives and obstetricians of the role of the midwife. Journal of Advanced Nursing 1:129–138

Watson N, Mander R 1995 Advertising infant formula in the maternity area. MIDIRS Midwifery Digest 5:338–341

Wilkerson V A 1984 The use of episiotomy in normal delivery. Midwives Chronicle 97:106–110

Williams S, Hepburn M, McIlwaine G 1985 Consumer view of epidural anaesthesia. Midwifery 1:32–36

Chapter 4

Routine antenatal HIV testing and its implications for informed consent

Rebecca Bennett

INTRODUCTION

Since 1994 there has been increasing optimism regarding the minimising of vertical HIV transmission from mother to child. In 1994 evidence emerged that zidovudine (ZDV) use during pregnancy, labour and after birth, could reduce the risk of HIV infection passed from mother to child from around 25% to around 8% (Connor et al 1994). More recent studies appear to indicate even further reductions using similar drug regimes combined with caesarean section delivery and not breastfeeding, perhaps reducing the risk of infection to as little as 2% (Mandelbrot et al 2001, McGowan et al 1999). While these treatments offered hope, many HIV positive women remained undiagnosed (Nicoll et al 1998).

In 1999 the United Kingdom (UK) government instructed health authorities to implement a policy of offering and recommending an HIV test to all pregnant women with the target of a 90% uptake of

HIV testing by pregnant women by 31 December 2002 (NHS Executive 1999 p 2). This approach was typical of those implemented in developed countries worldwide (Anonymous 1999, Centers for Disease Control and Prevention 1995).[1] The aim was that by encouraging universal antenatal HIV testing the rate of HIV transmission from mother to child could be dramatically reduced. As such these screening programmes are in line with an established tradition of such programmes that emphasise high rates of uptake in order to attempt to achieve their primary aim of reducing disease prevalence.

However, while HIV antenatal screening programmes may sit comfortably within a historical tradition of public health screening programmes, if they are to be compatible with modern ethical and legal practice it seems that they must take into account the need for informed consent by the patient to any diagnostic tests. Thus the UK antenatal HIV screening programme, and many like it, attempt to marry the public health aims of maximising uptake of testing with a commitment to respect the choices of patients by requiring informed consent before participation in screening occurs. This is no easy marriage. Maximising uptake of screening is, at least in some cases, incompatible with truly informed and voluntary consent.

It is midwives who are regularly left to implement these difficult policies, often with little in the way of guidance about how they should be approached. On the one hand health professionals are instructed to recommend the HIV test to all pregnant women to the point where the vast majority are expected to undergo the test (NHS Executive 1999, p 2) but at the same time aiming to ensure that:

> It is up to each woman to choose whether or not she is tested ... and she should not be pressurised into a decision either way. All testing for infections and conditions in pregnancy should be with the woman's knowledge, understanding and consent. (Department of Health/The Royal College of Midwives 1999 p 2)

Is it possible to uphold the rights of pregnant women to self-determined choices while achieving a high uptake of screening? If this is not possible, on which side should we place our emphasis? Is the need for fully voluntary informed consent more important

---

[1] This chapter concentrates on antenatal HIV testing and screening programmes in developed countries as, at the moment, treatment to minimise the risk of vertical transmission is not widely available. Also in some developing countries avoiding breast feeding and delivery by caesarean section is not seen as the most advisable option.

than a high uptake of HIV tests in pregnancy? Or is the possibility of providing HIV positive women with access to treatments that may prevent their child from being infected a sufficient reason to compromise fully voluntary informed consent in this instance? These questions must be explored in order that those implementing these programmes are not left in an impossible situation where the attempt to do the right thing pulls them in two different directions.

INFORMED CONSENT

It is generally accepted that competent individuals should be allowed to choose whether or not to have diagnostic tests, especially those that may indicate potentially serious conditions. While there may be temptations on the part of health professionals to test for conditions without the explicit informed consent of patients, such temptations are usually deemed unacceptably paternalistic (Gibson & Seaton 2000). It is normally assumed that the decision to undergo diagnostic tests, particularly those for diseases with serious consequences, should be a fully informed, freely chosen and carefully considered one. The General Medical Council (GMC) for instance stresses the importance of informed consent for any diagnostic test emphasising that

> [s]ome conditions, such as HIV, have serious social and financial, as well as medical, implications. In such cases you must make sure that the patient is given appropriate information about the implications of the test, and appropriate time to consider and discuss them. (GMC 1997 para 4)

This emphasis on informed consent for diagnostic procedures is, of course, in line with the current emphasis in health care on the rights of the patient to make autonomous choices about how and what treatment they wish to have. The principle of respect for autonomy is central to modern medical ethics and is often considered the most important principle in this area. Patient autonomy is increasingly and rightly perceived as a manifestation of the individual's rights of self-determination and privacy, universally regarded as a pillar of civil liberty, and this is reflected in legal and social policy as well as ethical doctrine.[2]

---

[2] See for example the European Convention on Human Rights, details of which can be found under Convention for the Protection of Human Rights and Fundamental Freedoms at http://conventions.coe.int/treaty/EN/cadreprincipal.htm

Thus, in most cases, it is important that an HIV test is undertaken on a voluntary basis, with the patient being given all the relevant information that is necessary to make such a decision, including the possible adverse consequences of being tested.

IS INFORMED CONSENT INCOMPATIBLE WITH A HIGH UPTAKE OF SCREENING?

While the GMC and other regulating bodies such as the American Medical Association insist that HIV testing should in most circumstances be freely chosen and preceded by explicit informed consent, antenatal HIV programmes often involve a significantly different approach to consent to testing. This approach to HIV testing in pregnancy has found its way into policy in many developed countries. Antenatal HIV programmes such as the one operated in the UK involve the routine offering and recommendation of an HIV test to all pregnant women, with the option of declining this offer of a test (NHS Executive 1999). It is perhaps not immediately clear that routine testing with the option of 'opting out' is incompatible with the standard requirement for informed consent, but for informed consent to have validity it must be freely given. The importance of gaining informed consent is grounded in the ethical principle of respecting the autonomous choices of individuals; thus informed consent is a safeguard protecting the choices of individuals. If the choice an individual makes is not freely taken—that is, it is arrived at as a result of some level of pressure or coercion—then it cannot truly be said to be the autonomous choice of that individual.

I will argue that there are four compelling reasons to suggest that gaining consent for routine HIV screening of this kind may often involve a level of coercion, albeit to a lesser extent than mandatory testing.

First, it is clear that programmes of routine testing are implemented in order to ensure that more people are tested than if the test had only been *offered*. In the UK in 1992 and 1994 the Department of Health issued recommendations that all pregnant women in high prevalence areas be offered an HIV test (Department of Health 1992, 1994). However, in 1996 it was estimated that only one in four of all the HIV positive women who gave birth in the UK knew that they were infected (Nicoll et al 1998). Of course this may have been as a result of a failure to implement these recommendations. However, research has shown that where testing is offered on an 'opt out' basis rather than an 'opt in' basis, a much greater uptake can be expected

(Le Gales et al 1990). One UK study compared an 'opt in' approach to antenatal HIV testing (where women had to make an active choice to be tested) to an 'opt out' study of the same test. It found that the uptake of 'opt out' testing (88%) was more than double the rate of the 'opt in' testing (35%). It is argued that even if some of the increase in uptake is due to increased knowledge and changing attitudes (the 'opt in' study was undertaken in 1996–7 and the 'opt out' study in 1998), the magnitude of the increase suggests that the approach to testing is significant (Simpson et al 1999).

Thus the fundamental aim of routine testing is to secure the testing of not only those women who would have elected to be tested, but also those women who would not have specifically chosen to be tested. If policy aims to ensure that high levels of uptake of routine testing are achieved, then it would seem that non-directive counselling will be impossible. Referring to antenatal screening programmes that involve routine testing for genetic disorders, Angus Clarke points out

> the very existence of a screening program amounts in effect to a recommendation that the testing thereby made available is a good thing. Health professionals and society would hardly establish and promote antenatal screening for Down's syndrome unless they wanted people to make use of it—the existence of such a program is an implicit, but powerful, recommendation to accept any screening offer made. Screening programs therefore, simply cannot be non-directive. Health professionals may respect the decisions of those who decline the offer of screening, not coercing them into compliance, but those who decide against participation will carry a label of social deviance unless great efforts have been made to avoid this. In practice, at least some of the personnel offering such tests are likely to regard those who decline screening as irritating, if not irresponsible, and to make this clear to their 'clients'. (Clarke 1998 p 401)

If one of the explicit targets of an antenatal HIV screening programme is to increase the number of women who are tested, then it seems inevitable that pressure will be put on women to accept the test. Midwives may even feel it is their duty to persuade women to accept the test and the benefits it may offer.

Second, for consent to be valid the individual must have adequate and accurate information. Providing only information that recommends testing and does not raise the possibilities of adverse consequences or discuss the effectiveness of treatments in some detail would seem to be inconsistent with freely given and informed consent. The GMC guidelines on consent to screening, for instance, emphasise that the standard level of information required for informed consent to other medical procedures should be given when testing as part of a screening programme, including a discussion of the uncertainties and risks attached to the programme (GMC 1998 para 34). It seems that, given the time constraints and the need to attain a high uptake of screening, it will be impossible in most cases for midwives providing antenatal care to give full and detailed information to all pregnant women about HIV and measures that can be taken to prevent vertical transmission. If the possible adverse consequences of testing and treatment were emphasised in pretest counselling this would seem likely to result in a lower uptake of testing than if only the positive consequences are emphasised. As an example of the information provided for pregnant women on this issue it is interesting to note the emotively titled Department of Health leaflet *Better for baby: HIV testing as part of your antenatal care* (Department of Health 1998). This leaflet is intended to be distributed to all pregnant women in Greater London and, as its title implies, strongly recommends the HIV test to pregnant women, offering a very one-sided view of the positive consequences of HIV testing.

Third, it had been suggested that one of the reasons why uptake of antenatal HIV testing is low on an 'opt in' basis is that some women are uncomfortable with making an active choice to be tested, as this choice may be perceived by others as an indication of high-risk behaviour (Simpson et al 1999). It has been suggested that making HIV screening in pregnancy routine and aiming for a high uptake will help to 'normalise' the test and remove this perceived stigmatisation (De Cock & Johnson 1998). However, even if encouraging routine testing of pregnant women does help to remove the stigma of the test, as well as allowing individuals to access antiretroviral drugs and even protect others from infection, this would be true of routine HIV testing of many other groups presenting for medical treatment. However, as we have already seen, there have been no attempts to routinely test other groups of patients for HIV. Diagnostic tests of these kinds in most other situations require explicit informed consent after counselling has provided information regarding not only the benefits but the possible consequences (including adverse consequences of testing).

Finally, the degree to which these kind of screening programmes limit pregnant women's autonomy does not seem to end at the routine test. If HIV testing is routinely recommended to pregnant women, then it is done in order that women will have access to the treatments and procedures that it is hoped will prevent the infection of their future child. If we accept that there is often a degree of coercion involved in the routine testing itself, and if the purpose of that testing is to enable the uptake of these risk-reducing measures for those who test positive, then it seems likely that women who test positive will feel under the same pressure to follow what might appear (however implicitly) the recommended path towards accepting these measures.

The implementation of any routine testing policy that aims for a high uptake cannot by its nature be non-directive and thus will not be compatible with authentic informed consent. Women in many cases will be directed towards being tested and accepting treatments and procedures they would not have elected to have chosen if the HIV test were offered in a non-directive way.

However, even if it is accepted that antenatal HIV screening programmes involve a degree of coercion that would generally be deemed unacceptable, this does not necessarily mean that such testing is ethically unacceptable. It may be that in certain circumstances it is entirely appropriate to recommend a particular course of action if there is strong evidence to suppose that this would be in the best interests of the patient. Health professionals routinely recommend (often in the strongest terms) that their patients stop smoking, cut down their alcohol intake, eat more healthily and take exercise. There is usually nothing 'non-directive' about the advice that is given on these sorts of subjects. Perhaps antenatal HIV testing is a similar situation where a certain level of coercion or persuasion is ethically acceptable in order to help the patient make a choice that reflects the evidence in favour of the benefits of HIV testing.

Further, while a testing regime that involves a level of coercion would infringe an individual's autonomy, it might be argued that this is ethically justified where this infringement is likely to protect a third party from serious harm. There may be strong arguments in favour of allowing individuals to make their own freely chosen decisions about diagnostic testing when the information that tests provide will only be pertinent to their own health state. Arguably the issues change dramatically when considering the related but distinct issue of whether individuals have a right to refuse tests which will provide information, not only about their own health state, but also that may allow them to protect others from harm.

Even the most liberal of commentators accept that it may be ethically justifiable to thwart an individual's autonomous choices in order to protect a third party from harm. This, of course, is the rationale behind traditional public health measures that, in extreme circumstances, allow the detention or enforced treatment of those with dangerous infectious diseases, in order to protect the wider public from infection.[3] So while individuals may, arguably, have the right to refuse information or treatment and in doing so risk their own health or happiness, it seems that this right is weakened by a risk to third parties from this decision. Thus it can be argued that there are justifiable exceptions to the right to individual autonomy in medical decision-making. The protection of others' physical well-being and their autonomy sometimes dictates that an individual's autonomous choices may be overridden. Hence it might be argued that some coercion is acceptable in screening programmes that aim to increase the uptake of HIV testing in an attempt to protect future children from HIV infection.

Is this the case? Is strongly recommending HIV testing for pregnant women analogous to strongly recommending smokers give up smoking or the obese lose weight? Or can it be justified on the same grounds as the enforced quarantine of those carrying highly infectious and serious communicable diseases?

The fundamental importance of the ethical and legal notion of respect for individual autonomy is well established in modern medicine. Given this, what is it that justifies directive counselling regarding unhealthy lifestyle choices such as overeating, smoking and excessive alcohol use, or justifies coercive measures with regard to highly infectious and dangerous diseases? In order for directive counselling to be acceptable it seems clear that the evidence to back up the advice must be sound. Coercive measures to prevent the transmission of dangerous infectious diseases must also be justified in part by evidence that these measures will be effective, and gain further justification (including perhaps far more coercive measures) from the fact that they are taken in order to attempt to prevent harm to third parties. So it seems that while attempts to strongly influence a patient's choices are generally deemed to be unjustified paternalism, when strong evidence is available to support the advice given and the level of coercion is relatively low (for instance, directive counselling), a strong case could be made that this coercion is justified because it is of such a low level. Further, higher levels of coercion may be justifiable where it is hoped that this coercion would protect third parties

---

[3] In the UK, for instance, the Public Health (Control of Diseases) Act 1984 empowers public health officers to act to prevent the spread of disease. The powers conferred by the Act and the Public Health (Infectious Diseases) Regulations 1988 permit the state to override virtually all individual liberties in the cause of protecting the community.

from harm. So, while it might be argued that in most other circumstances counselling for HIV testing should be non-directive it may be that if the evidence is strong that widespread antenatal HIV testing will prevent harm to future children, a level of coercion and lack of authentic informed consent may be justified in this instance.

EVALUATING THE EVIDENCE

Of the approximately 33 500 people living with HIV in the UK, about 30% remain undiagnosed. In 2000, of the 3654 new diagnoses of HIV reported, 52% were thought to be as a result of heterosexual sex. It has been estimated that 14 500 adults who had acquired their infection through heterosexual sex were living in the UK in 2000, and 6000 (41%) of these were unaware of their infection. It is thought that the highest proportion of undiagnosed HIV infection was in this category, with 48% of female heterosexuals and 36% of male heterosexuals unaware of their infection (Public Health Laboratory Service 2002b).

It is thought that there were 452 births to HIV infected women in the UK in 2000 (Public Health Laboratory Service 2002a). Since 1992 around 781 infants born in the UK have proved to be HIV positive probably as a result of vertical transmission of the virus from mother to infant (Public Health Laboratory Service 2002b). It is thought that three quarters of HIV positive women do not know that they are HIV positive at the time of their delivery (Nicoll et al 1998).

Vertical transmission of HIV is the transmission of the virus from an HIV positive mother to her child, either during pregnancy, birth or breastfeeding. In Europe there is thought to be a 15–20% chance of infection for a child born to an HIV infected woman if no specialist interventions are used—the figure is slightly higher in developing countries (Newell & Peckham 1993). The 1994 results of the Pediatric AIDS Clinical Trials Group (PACTG) protocol 076 which involved the use of ZDV during pregnancy, labour, and in the neonatal period showed a two thirds reduction, from 25.5% to 8.3%, in the risk of infection for the infant (Connor et al 1994). Around the same time as this influential ZDV trial, evidence emerged that, in a woman with established HIV infection, breastfeeding approximately doubles the risk of transmission (Newell & Peckham 1993) and that delivery by caesarean section may reduce the rate of vertical transmission (European Collaborative Study 1992). There is also evidence that avoidance of invasive procedures during pregnancy and labour may help reduce the risk of transmission (European Collaborative Study 1991). This evidence has been substantiated and strengthened by subsequent trials. More recent preliminary data appear to indicate that use of such risk-reducing regimes by HIV positive pregnant women may be associated with a further decrease in risk of vertical transmission to 2% or less (Mandelbrot et al 2001, McGowan et al 1999).

The hope is that the UK programme of routine antenatal HIV screening, if it achieves the target of increasing HIV test uptake to 90% of all pregnant women in the UK 'will result in 80% reduction in the number of children with HIV acquired from an infected mother during pregnancy, birth or through breastfeeding' (NHS Executive 1999 p 2). As we have seen, in 2000 it was estimated that around 450 HIV positive women will give birth in the UK each year (Public Health Laboratory Service 2002a). On the evidence collected it seems that where only an 'opt in' antenatal HIV testing policy exists we can expect only a quarter of these 450 women to be aware of their infection (Nicoll et al 1998). If we accept that the transmission rate is around 2% where these treatments and procedures are adhered to, and around 20% where they are not, then if 25% of these 450 women who are aware of their HIV status are tested and accept treatment but 75% do not, it can be predicted that 69.75 of the children born to these 450 women will be infected with the virus. If, however, 90% of the 450 women are tested and accept a drug regime, a caesarean section and do not breastfeed, it can be predicted that only 17.1 of the children will become infected with HIV. Thus, if the UK government's programme of antenatal HIV screening succeeds in reaching its uptake target of 90%, and if all women who test positive accept the treatments offered, it can be estimated that this may prevent 52.65 children becoming infected with HIV in the UK per year.

This would seem to provide the strong evidence that is generally needed to justify instances of deviation from the usual doctrine of respect for patient autonomy. A result of this magnitude in terms of infection avoided would seem to provide strong justification for routine antenatal screening programmes even if they involve a level of coercion that in other areas of health care would be deemed ethically unacceptable. But is this an accurate picture of the evidence, and even if it is accurate, is coercive testing necessarily the best option? There are a number of other issues that deserve our consideration if we are to analyse this issue effectively.

COMPLIANCE

First, the predictions given assume that all those who test positive will wish to and will be able to accept the risk-reducing treatments/

procedures that offer this hope of minimising vertical transmission rates. The drug regime recommended in these circumstances can be very difficult to maintain. Taking ZDV can cause nausea (Rabaud et al 2001) and as pregnant women may already be nauseous this can make compliance with the regime even more difficult (IAPAC 2001). Adherence to the neonatal drug regime may also be difficult. The current prophylaxis for full-term HIV exposed newborns involves a 6-week course of oral ZDV in 2 mg doses 4 times a day (Centers for Disease Control and Prevention 1994). This intensive regime will often be coupled with the distress that may have been caused by the diagnosis of HIV and concerning the welfare of the infant (Demas et al 2002). Caesarean section poses a much greater risk to women than vaginal delivery, and greater risk still to those whose immune systems may be compromised by HIV infection, and thus may not be accepted readily by the women concerned (Stringer et al 1999). If women fail to comply with the treatments and procedures offered, then the number of infants protected from HIV infection will decrease.

It has been suggested that 'compliance with medical care is likely to be greatest when the woman feels she has made an informed decision regarding HIV testing and has a relationship of respect and trust with her health care provider' (Mofenson 2000 p 7). If this is correct then it seems that a coercive antenatal HIV screening programme will only be detrimental to the already difficult issue of compliance.

SAFETY

If we accept that the vertical transmission rate without specialist intervention will be around 20%, then it can be expected that 80% of children born to HIV infected women will not be infected even if their mothers' HIV status remains unknown. Thus it seems that in order to prevent infection in 52.65 children a year, 307.35 women have to undergo arguably unnecessary caesarean sections and ZDV use, while 307.35 children are exposed to the extra risks involved in ZDV use and are denied the benefits of breastfeeding. These women thus have an increased risk of complications due to caesarean delivery and there may be worries that ZDV use in pregnancy and administering ZDV to infants after birth may have, as yet, undisclosed complications. Animal models have suggested that adverse consequences of ZDV use may be possible (Olivero et al 1997, Poirier et al 1999). At the moment it appears that short-term ZDV use for infants is safe, although long-term data are not yet available (Culnane et al 1999, Hanson et al 1999).

AREAS OF LOW INCIDENCE

National unlinked anonymous monitoring of the prevalence of HIV infection in pregnant women began in 1988 and since 1992 the survey has covered approximately 70% of the UK. The results of this unlinked monitoring have indicated that outside London the prevalence of HIV infection among women giving birth to live-born infants has remained low. In England in the first 6 months of 2001 there were 64 births to HIV infected women (4.0 per 10 000 women); in Scotland, 16 HIV infected women gave birth to live-born infants in 2001 (3.0 per 10 000); and in at least one area no HIV positive pregnant women were identified (Public Health Laboratory Service 2001, 2002a). In many low incidence areas 90% uptake of the HIV test in pregnancy will not prevent any infants from becoming infected, may cause a large number of women distress at a difficult time and may even result in some false positive test results, as these are relatively much more likely in areas of low prevalence.

A CLEAR PICTURE OF INFECTION?

Following infection with HIV there is an initial period during which antibodies to the virus have not been produced—a 'window period' that can last for 8 to 10 weeks. If an infected individual is tested for HIV antibodies during this period the result will be negative. Antenatal HIV testing is typically offered early in a pregnancy, so unless the HIV test is repeated later on in the pregnancy, it seems that a number of newly infected women will receive a false negative result.

ERODING OF PATIENT AUTONOMY FOR PREGNANT WOMEN?

If antenatal HIV screening programmes involve the erosion of pregnant women's autonomous choices in this area, this erosion of autonomy is an attempt to benefit the resulting child. If this is accepted as a justified infringement of autonomy, then it may be argued that other coercive measures can be justified for similar reasons. If preventing harm to future children is sufficient justification for infringing pregnant women's autonomy then it may be possible that this justification will be used, not only to sanction the relatively noninvasive methods of directive counselling for HIV testing and treatment, but also far more invasive infringements.

There have already been calls to make antenatal HIV testing mandatory (Rovner 1996) and there are now proposals that those women who evade testing by not presenting for antenatal care should be tested for HIV when they present in labour (Kane 1999). Could establishing the acceptance of coercion in order to prevent harm to infants in the case of antenatal HIV screening pave the way for enforced antenatal HIV testing or even enforced treatment such as caesarean section? High profile cases which involve attempts to legally enforce caesarean section deliveries in labour have attempted to justify this enforced treatment by appealing to the welfare of the child who will be born (Draper 1996). While we may think that 'low level' coercion to persuade women to be tested for HIV is acceptable, what if this leads to more dramatic infringements of women's autonomy, not just with regard to HIV but to any possible harms to unborn children, would we find this as acceptable? It seems the same reasoning applies (see Chapters 1 and 2).

CONCLUSIONS

Midwives and other health professionals who are left to implement antenatal HIV screening programmes are often put in an impossible position. Where screening programmes aim for a high uptake of HIV testing then there will inevitably be conflict between the need to secure this high uptake and the need to uphold the autonomous choices of the women involved. On the one hand, aiming to identify as many HIV positive pregnant women as possible when there is good evidence that this diagnosis may enable these women to protect their children from HIV infection is clearly laudable. On the other hand, we normally assume that it is important to protect every competent individual's right to have their autonomy respected by being enabled to make freely chosen and fully informed choices about their futures. How the information about antenatal screening is given will undoubtedly have an effect on both the uptake of the test and the authenticity of the consent given (Banatvala & Chrystie 1994, Simpson et al 1988). If a high uptake is to be achieved, the information given should emphasise the benefits of screening and pressure in the form of directive counselling must be applied. If the counselling given is truly non-directive and accurate, and balanced information is given which discusses the possible adverse consequences of testing, this will enable women to make freely chosen informed decisions about their treatment but is likely to produce more rejections of the HIV test than a more directive approach.

The present situation regarding antenatal screening programmes like that implemented in the UK is unsatisfactory. It is often left to those implementing the screening programmes to decide which is the most important outcome—a high uptake of the HIV test or ensuring fully informed choice—and to pitch the information and counselling given accordingly. This is an extremely complex and difficult issue and needs to be debated in a more transparent way in order to arrive at a more satisfactory situation.

Antenatal HIV screening programmes have been implemented for extremely good reasons but have often tried to marry two commendable but often incompatible aims. If, as I have argued, succeeding in producing a high uptake of HIV screening while also succeeding in enabling truly informed choices is often impossible, then a decision has to be made. Should we allow a degree of coercion or pressure to be put on to pregnant women in order to procure a high uptake of HIV testing, or should we protect informed consent from any erosion? Whatever we choose to do, this choice needs to be transparent and explicit and the reasons behind it stated and debated. At present we are left with a well-intentioned fudge where a smoke screen that looks like informed consent but is not truly informed consent conceals levels of coercion that are not deemed acceptable in many other areas of medical testing or treatment. If a compelling case can be made that this coercion is justifiable given the available evidence, even though it may go against the usual insistence on respect for individual autonomy, then there should be no reason to disguise this behind a smoke screen. This justification and aim of screening should be made clear.

In attempting to produce such a compelling case all the aspects of this issue need to be considered extremely carefully. A strong case would need to establish why this approach would be preferable to one that resisted coercion. Difficult questions would need to be addressed. Can this infringement of pregnant women's autonomy be prevented from slipping into more invasive infringements such as enforced treatment and caesarean section based on the same grounds? Will a screening programme which contains a level of coercion but does not enforce treatment have better results in terms of minimising vertical transmission than a screening programme that aims for a high uptake of accurate information rather than testing?

Antenatal screening programmes that aim for a high uptake of testing and treatment and thus often involve a degree of coercion, may not produce the level of benefits that is predicted. Not all HIV positive pregnant women will be identified, not all women will adhere to the treatments, there may be some complications arising from the drug regimes and the relationship between midwife and woman may suffer a loss of trust. Before resorting to coercive screening programmes it is important to consider carefully the efficacy of the alternatives. By implementing a policy of routine antenatal HIV counselling (with testing as a truly voluntary option), it would be hoped that all pregnant women could receive balanced information about HIV, accurately informing them of the treatments available both for themselves and for their children. While this may result in a lower uptake of testing, it may be that by upholding women's autonomy and providing accurate information in a balanced way, women will not only be encouraged to be tested for HIV but also may even be more likely to accept treatments offered. Providing information about HIV in this non-coercive atmosphere may also allow women access to counselling about high-risk behaviours and may, therefore, help prevent vertical transmission by reducing the increase of women who become infected with HIV in the first place.

References

[Anonymous] 1999 Antenatal HIV testing in Europe. Eurosurveillance Weekly 34. Online. Available: www.eurosurv.org/1999/990819.html 19 August

Banatvala J E, Chrystie I L 1994 HIV Screening in pregnancy: UK lags. Lancet 343:1113–1114

Centers for Disease Control and Prevention 1994 Recommendations of the US Public Health Service task force on the use of zidovudine to reduce perinatal transmission of human immunodeficiency virus. Morbidity and Mortality Weekly Report 43 (RR-11):1–20

Centers for Disease Control and Prevention 1995 Recommendations for HIV counseling and testing for pregnant women. Morbidity and Mortality Weekly Report 44 (RR-07): 1–15

Clarke A 1998 Genetic counselling. In: Chadwick R (ed) Encyclopaedia of applied ethics, volume 2. Academic Press, San Diego

Connor E M, Sperling M D, Gelber R et al 1994 Reduction of maternal–infant transmission of human immunodeficiency virus type 1 with zidovudine treatment. New England Journal of Medicine 331:1173–1179

Culnane M, Fowler M, Lee S S 1999 Lack of long-term effects of in utero exposure to zidovudine among uninfected children born to HIV-infected women. Journal of the American Medical Association 281:151–157

De Cock K M, Johnson A M 1998 From exceptionalism to normalisation: a reappraisal of attitudes and practices around HIV testing. British Medical Journal 316:290–293

Demas P A, Webber M P, Schoenbaum E E et al 2002 Maternal adherence to the zidovudine regimen for HIV-exposed infants to prevent HIV infection: a preliminary study. Pediatrics 110 (3). Online. Available: www.pediatrics.org/cgi/content/full/110/3/e35

Department of Health 1992 Department of Health guidance PL/CO(92)5, appendix 2: guidelines for offering voluntary named HIV testing to women receiving antenatal care. Department of Health, London

Department of Health 1994 Department of Health guidance PL/CO (94) guidelines for offering voluntary named HIV antibody testing to women receiving antenatal care. Department of Health, London

Department of Health 1998 Better for baby: HIV testing as part of your antenatal care PL/CO(98)4, produced by the Expert Advisory Group on AIDS. Online. Available: http://www.doh.gov.uk/eaga/betterbaby.htm

Department of Health/The Royal College of Midwives 1999 HIV testing in pregnancy: helping women choose. Information for Midwives. Online. Available: http://www.rcm.org.uk

Draper H 1996 Women, forced caesareans and antenatal responsibilities. Journal of Medical Ethics 22:327–333

European Collaborative Study 1991 Children born to women with HIV-1 infection: natural history and risk of transmission. Lancet 337:253–260

European Collaborative Study 1992 Risk factors for mother-to-child transmission of HIV-1. Lancet 339:1007–1012

General Medical Council 1997 Serious communicable diseases: guidance to doctors. Online. Available: http://www.gmc-uk.org/global_sections/sitemap_frameset.htm

General Medical Council 1998 Seeking patients' consent: the ethical considerations. Online. Available: http://www.gmc-uk.org/standards

Gibson G J, Seaton A 2000 GMC's advice in serious communicable diseases. British Medical Journal 320:1727

Hanson I C, Antonelli T A, Sperling R S 1999 Lack of tumors in infants with perinatal HIV-1 exposure and fetal/neonatal exposure to zidovudine. Journal of Acquired Immune Deficiency Syndromes and Human Retrovirology 463–467

International Association of Physicians in AIDS Care (IAPAC) 2001 Considerations for antiretroviral therapy in the HIV-infected woman. IAPAC Monthly: Guidelines for the use of antiretroviral agents in HIV infected adults and adolescents Supplement 7 (1): S29. Online. Available: http://www.iapac.org/Text/pdf/Guidelines%203_01.pdf

Kane B 1999 Rapid testing for HIV: why so fast? Annals of Internal Medicine 131:481–483

Le Gales C, Moatti J P and The Paris-Tours study group of antenatal transmission of HIV 1990 Cost effectiveness of HIV screening of pregnant women in hospital in the Paris area. European Journal of Obstetrics & Gynecology and Reproductive Biology 37:25–33

McGowan J P, Crane M, Wiznia A A et al 1999 Combination antiretroviral therapy in human immunodeficiency virus-infected pregnant women. Obstetetrics and Gynecology 94:641–646

Mandelbrot L, Landreau-Mascaro A, Rekacewicz C et al 2001 Lamivudine-zidovudine combination for prevention of maternal–infant transmission of HIV-1. Journal of the American Medical Association 285:2083–2093

Mofenson L M and the Committee on Pediatric AIDS 2000 Technical report: perinatal human immunodeficiency virus testing and prevention of transmission. Commission on Pediatric Aids (review). Pediatrics 106(6):E88. Online. Available: http://www.pediatrics.org/cgi/content/full/106/6/e88

Newell M L, Peckham C S 1993 Risk factors for vertical transmission and early markers of HIV-1 infection in children. AIDS 7:S591–597

NHS Executive 1999 Reducing mother to baby transmission of HIV. Health Service Circular HSC 1999/183. Online. Available: http://www.doh.gov.uk/coinh/htm 13 August

Nicoll A, McGarrigle C, Brady A R et al 1998 Epidemiology and detection of HIV-1 among pregnant women in the United Kingdom: results from national surveillance 1988–96. British Medical Journal 316 (7127):253–258

Olivero O A, Anderson L M, Diwan B A 1997 Transplacental effect of 3'-azido-2',3'-dideoxythymidine (AZT): tumorigenicity in mice and genotoxicity in mice and monkeys. Journal of the National Cancer Institute 89:1602–1608

Poirier M C, Patterson T A, Slikker W, Olivero O A 1999 Incorporation of 3'-azido-2',3'-deoxythymidine (AZT) into fetal DNA and fetal tissue distribution of drug after infusion of pregnant late-term rhesus macaques with a human-equivalent AZT dose. Journal of Acquired Immune Deficiency Syndromes and Human Retrovirology 22:477–483

Public Health Laboratory Service News Bulletin 2001 Infectious diseases in the news—01 June 2001: recent news stories: key points. Online. Available: http://www.phls.co.uk/news/bulletins/2001id.htm

Public Health Laboratory Service 2002a HIV infection in women giving birth in the United Kingdom—trends in prevalence and proportions diagnosed to the end of June 2001 12 (17). Online. Available: http://www.phls.org.uk/publications/cdr/archive02/hivarchive02.html#AIDS1702 25 April

Public Health Laboratory Service 2002b AIDS and HIV infection in the United Kingdom: monthly report—January 2002 12 (5). Online. Available: http://www.phls.org.uk/publications/cdr/archive02/hivarchive02.html 31 January

Rabaud C, Bevilacqua S, Beguinot I et al 2001 Tolerability of postexposure prophylaxis with zidovudine, lamivudine, and nelfinavir for human immunodeficiency virus infection. Clinical Infectious Diseases 32(10):1494

Rovner J 1996 US specialists object to AMA's call for mandatory testing. The Lancet 348 (9023):330

Simpson W M, Johnston F, Boyd F M et al 1988 Uptake and acceptability of antenatal HIV testing: randomised controlled trial of different methods of offering the test. British Medical Journal 316:262–316

Simpson W M, Johnstone F D, Goldberg D J et al 1999 Antenatal HIV testing: assessment of a routine voluntary approach. British Medical Journal 318:1660–1661

Stringer S A, Rouse D J, Goldenberg R L 1999 Prophylactic cesarean delivery for the prevention of perinatal human immunodeficiency virus transmission: the case for restraint. Journal of the American Medical Association 281:1946–1949

Chapter 5

Risk and normality in the maternity services

Soo Downe

INTRODUCTION

It is not uncommon for midwives to pronounce themselves 'experts in normal childbirth'. This assertion goes largely unchallenged and is seen as a matter of some pride—even as a fundamental statement of identity. In using it, it is assumed that the term 'normality' does not need explanation. However, normality is not a fixed concept; it is socially defined and changes over time. It was once perfectly normal to believe that the earth was flat and those who thought otherwise were blasphemers; that the body was controlled by humours; and that blood letting was good for the sick. Contemporary western culture has rejected these beliefs—indeed, for most people in the modern world, such ideas would be considered ludicrous. However, contemporary society is less willing to consider how quickly knowledge and knowledge bases have changed within the lifetimes of individuals, or to reflect on the possibility that some current firmly fixed beliefs will seem quaint in even half a century's time.

Definitions of normality are increasingly filtered through scientific and technological advances. These advances prioritise research based on pathology, and on the belief that adverse outcomes can be minimised through scientific knowledge. As a consequence, abnormality is increasingly defined as a deviation from the average, with the potential for pathology, rather than as a pathological entity in its own right. This phenomenon is having two major effects. First, and most importantly, it forces increasing numbers of women into widely defined risk groups on the grounds that a deviation from the average is an abnormality until proven otherwise. Second, it causes the practice of midwifery to be ever more narrowly circumscribed.

This chapter seeks to examine the impact of an increasingly risk-based philosophy on the nature of normality in childbirth in the UK in the early 21st century. In the process it explores three applications of the concept of normality: beliefs about the nature of pregnancy and birth; decisions about the normality of the fetus; and beliefs about whether the behaviour of the pregnant woman fits the norms of society. Implications for users of maternity services are considered. The impact of technological screening on beliefs about normality are explored, and finally the implications of these changes for the midwifery profession and its role in childbirth are highlighted.

APPLICATION OF RISK ASSESSMENT

Risk assessment has been a regular feature of maternity care, albeit implicitly, for many years. It is in the area of antenatal care that most effort has been focused, attempting prospectively to define the nature of risk. Many formal risk scoring systems utilise large databases of retrospective data and logistic regression techniques to identify women at risk. The idea is that if enough pieces of information about women are collected, and if enough is known about their outcomes in pregnancy and labour, predictions can be made about likely outcomes for other women with similar characteristics. Prophylactic intervention can then be instigated to reduce morbidity and mortality in those groups with the highest statistical risk. However, as Enkin et al (2000) point out, there are many pitfalls with this type of data collection, not least in defining the relevant clinical data in the first place. Furthermore, the choice of abnormal outcome used in assessing risk is crucial. Often this is perinatal mortality, but the problem with this measure is that it is so rare that large numbers of women need to receive an intervention in order to decrease mortality by very small amounts. In addition, any observed decrease may itself be due to a number of factors that are not amenable to manipulation by obstetric interventions. The scoring system then fails the two fundamental requirements of a screening test; first that it accurately discriminates between those who are and who are not at high risk, and second, that the findings resulting from its use can affect care management and, crucially, 'help our patient reach her goals' (Sackett 2000 p 81).

The addition of weighted scales and cumulative scores only serves to compound these factors. The 1958 perinatal mortality survey and the consequent longitudinal National Child Development Study were probably some of the earliest sets of data used to assess risk (Butler et al 1969). In 1970 the British Births Survey was published. This proposed a scoring system for risk based on the 1958 data (Chamberlain et al 1978). The idea was that a cumulative score, which was weighted for the contribution of particular factors, would be a good predictor of outcome. Although these data now relate to a previous generation of women the factors identified form the basis of many formal and informal risk assessment systems today (Campbell 1999). For this reason, it is instructive to look in some detail at the way this particular system was constructed, and at some of the implications of its application.

The following comprised the antenatal prediction scoring system (see Table 5.1):

Risk status was defined as follows:

- 0–2: low
- 3–7: median
- 8+ : high.

Table 5.1 suggests that, all other things being equal, a woman having her second baby after a previous spontaneous abortion is at a fourfold greater risk of perinatal mortality in the current pregnancy than a woman who has not had a miscarriage. Given the fact that current predictions put the rate of miscarriage at 1 in 7 pregnancies (Enkin et al 2000), this risk scoring alone would put many women into the median risk group. It must be acknowledged that, in 1958, known miscarriages would probably have been at a later gestation than those currently diagnosed after very early pregnancy tests. The relative insensitivity of the scoring system cannot, however, differentiate between an early and a late miscarriage, with their very different aetiology, and therefore its application (and the interventions that could be imposed as a result of its application) may not be appropriate for the individual. Spontaneous abortion due to a lethal dominant chromosomal abnormality may well be a good predictor of subsequent perinatal risk, but an unexplained loss at 6 weeks probably would not be.

Table 5.1   British Births Survey. Antenatal risk scoring system

Factor	Score
Maternal age	
20–29	0
<20 and 30–34	1
35 and older	2
Parity	
1 and 2	0
0 and 3	1
4 and over	2
Social class	
I and II	0
III	1
IV and V and unemployed	2
Unsupported mothers (single, separated, divorced, widowed)	2
Previous obstetric performance	
Stillbirth	4
Neonatal death	4
Abortion	4
Caesarean section	4
Medical history	
Hypertension (BP 140/90 or more before 20 weeks' gestation)	4
Diabetes	4

EFFECTS ON WOMEN

Risk systems are population-, not person-, specific. For example, in the British Births Survey (Chamberlain et al 1978), a 36-year-old social class one woman with no pre-existing disease, who had planned the pregnancy, who swam regularly and ate healthily, but who had one previous miscarriage at 8 weeks, and was 5 feet 1 inch tall would score 8 and be in the high risk group. With her in the high risk group could be a woman of the same age and class who was 5 feet 2 inches tall, but who smoked 40 cigarettes a day, often binge-drank, never took any exercise, and whose pregnancy was completely unplanned and unwanted. Further, as far as individual women are concerned, risk scoring is of no benefit if something cannot be done to modify the risk. In the case of events occurring before the current pregnancy (such as past obstetric history) or of present physiological data (such as maternal height), modifications cannot be made.

Even though formal risk scoring is not often used now, informal assessment of risk is a part of everyday practice. Where formal risk scores are used, as in criteria for booking women into different places of birth, there appears to be no consistency between different maternity services in the constituents of the risk system (Campbell 1999).

Handwerker (1994) discusses the ways in which the application of 'high risk' labels leads to the censoring of pregnant women who fail to comply with medical advice. The application of such risk markers, if pushed to their logical conclusion, results in judging as antisocial, or even criminal, women who are unable or unwilling to act on the clinical predictions derived from them. A recent example involved a woman who was known to be HIV positive, and who refused to consent to HIV testing for her baby, on the basis of her own reading of the current research evidence (Dodd 1999). The consequent court order against her forced her and her family into hiding. Her insistence on normalising her situation was seen as criminal, and as tantamount to child abuse, since it contradicted assumptions about what was seen as being properly in the realm of abnormality, and thus under medical control. Similar cases have been reported elsewhere (Wolf et al 2001).

This application of the concept of risk is an illustration of a potential imbalance between the attempt to effect benevolence for the baby while, at the same time, violating the principle of non-maleficence for the mother. Its most extreme consequences are court-ordered caesarean sections against the will of pregnant women or even long-term imprisonment of drug-using women in pregnancy. These policies are based on an assumption that risk is the same as inevitable pathology, and on a failure to assess the relative stressors and values of women and families in widely different cultures.

Cross-cultural assumptions also affect women's experience of the allocation of risk. The effect of maternal age is a case in point. The researchers analysing the National Child Development Study (Butler et al 1969) varied their categorisation of age, but the most frequent allocation gave a low risk of adverse outcomes to the babies of women in the 20–29-year-old group, a median risk to those in the 30–34 group and a high risk to the over 35 group. This perception of risk obtains still today, although it is increasingly being questioned as the average age of childbearing women creeps upwards. While researchers are still concluding that maternal age is associated with increased risks (Rosenthal & Paterson-Brown 1998), an earlier study designed to control for confounders demonstrated that, although intervention rates were universally higher in nulliparous women over 35 compared with younger matched controls, neonatal outcomes were not worse (Edge & Laros 1993). This may demonstrate that intervention works in minimising pre-existing risk. However, Edge and Laros (1993) undertook a regression analysis of matched cases and controls, and found that the higher caesarean section rate amid the over-35s was only partially explained by obvious complications. This begs the question of cause and effect. Is the greater level of intervention found in older childbearing women influencing the outcome positively, or are high intervention rates a function of the labelling of abnormality, with no improvement in the outcomes? It may well be that, historically, older women were more at risk, either through grand multiparity, or because of poorly controlled underlying disease (such as diabetes) which caused subfertility and therefore delayed childbearing. This assumption of underlying pathology is, however, less relevant in the early 21st century as more women choose to have babies later, fewer have large families and maternal disease is better controlled.

While it may be assumed that the consequences of over-application of risk scoring are most evident in ever increasing rates of caesarean section (Thomas & Paranjothy 2001) there is also evidence that most women who had a so-called 'normal' birth have in fact experienced a number of interventions (Downe et al 2001). The maternal, fetal and infant consequences of this hidden application of just-in-case intervention remains to be fully researched.

In summary, the benefits and iatrogenic drawbacks of risk-scoring are still to be established:

> ... the potential benefits of risk scoring have been widely publicised, but the potential harm is rarely mentioned. Such harm can result from unwarranted intrusion in women's private lives, from superfluous interventions and treatments, from creating unnecessary stress and anxiety, and from allocation of scarce resources to areas where they are not needed. (Enkin et al 2000 p 52)

TECHNOLOGICAL SCREENING

The focus has now shifted from the retrospective analysis of risk in the general population to the discovery of physiological markers of variants in the individual. It may seem, as we gather increasing information about the microscopic changes in the body of a pregnant woman and that of her fetus, that we have at last obtained the skills and knowledge to fully understand the deviations from the normal and can to begin to give women an individualised assessment of risk. However, it appears that even (and perhaps especially) in this field our knowledge is at best partial and its application contentious. The development of ever more powerful technology carries the potential to see what has not previously been seen—without knowledge about its relative normality. When new markers are identified, it is not always clear whether they are merely non-suspicious variants seen only in a minority, or if they are true deviations. If the assumption is made that what is seen in the majority of cases is the normal, then what is seen in the minority of cases becomes abnormal until proven otherwise.

Most researchers developing tests understand the necessity of maximum sensitivity (the ability to detect all the problems) and specificity (the ability to detect only the problems and to avoid the discovery of 'problems' where none in fact exist). Lilford et al (1983) in discussing the value of the placental lactogen test in predicting the risk of fetal growth retardation, illustrate the point that what is normal and what is abnormal is, on occasion, a matter of debate and entails a trade-off between sensitivity and specificity for a particular marker or test: 'Clinical interpretation of any biochemical test depends on the definition of a cut-off point … above or below which the patient is considered "abnormal" for the purposes of subsequent decision making' (Lilford et al 1983 p 511). It is not, therefore, an absolute indicator of when things will go wrong for mother and baby—but merely a marker for the extreme finding, which may, in fact, be perfectly benign.

It could be argued that if a test is sensitive and specific, if it is testing for a problem that is of real concern to the individual as well as to society, and if there is a real chance of avoiding or eradicating the problem without causing harm, then that test passes, in an ethical sense, the rule of beneficence. However, tests should also pass the test of non-maleficence and it is here that the problem arises. If these criteria are not satisfied—that is, if a test does not pick up all those with the problem, or if it identifies some as having a problem when they do not, or if the problem is not seen as such by the individual or by society until the test makes it obvious, or if there is not a harm-free solution to the problem—one may begin to ask whether the test itself risks becoming the cause of iatrogenic distress.

Sophisticated screening and scanning both reveal and define our experience of the abnormal. At the extreme, this concept encompasses the fetus itself. The relatively subjective decisions made when choosing the cut-off point for 'high risk' are crucial in screening tests for fetal abnormality, where the chosen cut-off point has major psychological and physical implications for the woman, the fetus and their family. There is now a very large body of evidence relating to the use of tests and scans to identify the abnormal fetus— but very little literature on either the ethics of such definitions and their consequences, or on the dividing line between normality and abnormality in this context.

One of the key ethical problems at the heart of this explosion of screening and scanning is that the only cure for the supposedly abnormal child is the termination of the pregnancy (see Chapter 8). The psychological impact of this on parents and family—the potential maleficence—is as yet extremely poorly measured, let alone compared with the psychosocial consequences of parenting a child with profound impairments. The ethical impact of the definition of abnormality in this area is as yet unexplored. How far will society go in assuming abnormality and in insisting on termination, or in refusing to support an abnormal child that the parents knowingly decide not to terminate? Will the elimination of the more obvious abnormalities render currently acceptable deviations from the average unacceptable in the future? Who decides what is abnormal when the prognosis for any individual fetus (even with a known chromosomal abnormality) is impossible to predict? It is important to note that even the development of such technology changes the experience of pregnancy itself for all women into one of potential abnormality, rather than anticipated normality (Rothman 1994), and the impact of this revolution is yet to be assessed.

> Costs are not wholly financial, and it is equally important to weigh the human costs. Although screening programs may bring reassurance to some women who are tested, for others they may generate anxiety by merely raising the question of abnormality. The consequences of erroneous diagnoses must be a matter for particularly careful consideration. (Daker & Bobrow 1989 p 31)

Arney (1982), a sociologist, examined the phenomenon of the rise and dominance of obstetrics in Europe and America, differentiating three periods of development. The first and second periods are discussed in the following section. He proposes that, currently, a third phase of obstetrics exists, which he calls the monitoring period.

He claims that this is characterised by a nominally team approach to maternity care, with the obstetrician in the role of 'expert', dealing with the physiological, and the midwife allied with the women in the psychological sphere of care giving. The most interesting aspect of this analysis is the recognition that, first, the technology needed for increasingly precise monitoring is out of the control of the practitioners involved, and second, that the extension of monitoring implies that it scrutinises every facet of the women's life and makes a judgement on it. This aspect is particularly acute, and the ethical problems particularly complex, when such scrutiny is deemed to put mother and child into conflict. The imprisoning of pregnant drug-using women in some states of America, or the imposition of court-ordered caesarean sections are the most extreme examples of the moral complexities which arise from the societal imposition of the concept of 'normality' on to individuals within that society. It is at this moral junction that the development of ever more complex technologies for observing new and uninterpretable phenomena has its greatest potential for iatrogenic impact both in terms of physical damage (when the true meaning of the findings are not known and intervention causes harm) and psychologically (when the general values of society conflict with the specific, even if unrecognised, values of the individual).

EFFECTS ON MIDWIFERY

Arney's (1982) first two phases of obstetrics are informative in indicating how midwifery has evolved over the last few centuries. In his view, the first phase was the preprofessional period, characterised by a symbiosis between barber surgeons and midwives, with midwives dealing with the normal, and barber surgeons the abnormal. The next phase, the so-called professional period, marginalised the midwives, and perceived all births as having a pathological potential. He states that

> The rational approach to childbirth which crossed the channel into Britain undermined the symbolic basis of the traditional midwives' practice by blurring the demarcation between 'normal' and 'abnormal' births ... This reformulation of the ideological basis of midwifery was essential to the ultimate success of male midwives in their struggle against women practitioners. (Arney 1982 p 25)

He goes on crucially to state that: '[t]he midwife had control ... over the distinction between normal and abnormal, and it was on the control of this distinction that her power rested' (Arney 1982 p 25). He observes that the new theory of 'abnormality' did not have a clear application. It was enough to introduce the concepts, and to define the parameters, to effect the removal of power from midwives and essentially to cause the reallocation of the management of women whose bodies did not conform to a norm.

Professional demarcation around the birth of a breech baby serves as an example. In 1958, the Myles *Textbook for Midwives* clearly locates breech presentation under malpresentation in the section entitled 'Abnormal labour' and states that a doctor should be informed if the breech persists beyond 32 weeks gestation, mainly in order to attempt an external cephalic version. The potential complications arising from a breech delivery are noted, and the comment is made that:

> ...although midwives are permitted by the Central Midwives Board to undertake the delivery of breech presentations at home, they would be well advised only to do so in an emergency. The opinion of most obstetricians is that, because of the risks to the foetus, multiparae as well as primiparae should be delivered in hospital where expert assistance is available. (Myles 1958 p 359)

However, the textbook continues to assume that it will be the midwife who attends these births, even in the complex situation where the baby's legs are extended (Myles 1958 p 367). It is also acknowledged that in even more difficult situations (such as extended arm or head) the midwife may be in attendance at a home birth, and that she therefore needs to be taught how to manage the situation. In this case, such births are still seen to be in the domain of the midwife. Although textbooks being produced today continue to instruct midwives in the techniques associated with breech births (Bennett & Brown 1999), it is increasingly uncommon for midwives to do so on their own responsibility, if at all. This fact is picked up by the midwives interviewed by Leap & Hunter (1993), in their analysis of the work of midwives and handywomen who began practising in the 1920s and 1930s. They note that 'although a breech birth at home would be considered an emergency nowadays, in pre-NHS days such births were considered normal' (p 178). Edie B, one of the midwives interviewed, said: 'oh, I used to love delivering breeches. The breech births were so easy ... And we never used to have any problems with them' (p 179).

To assist a woman in a breech birth was by no means an unfamiliar activity to midwives at home or in hospital until comparatively

Table 5.2 British Births Survey. Length of
labour risk score

Duration of labour	Score
Duration of first stage of labour:	
<12 hours	0
12–24 hours	1
24 hours +	2

recently. Now most midwives consider it to be inadvisable, a view
reinforced by the publication of the results of the Term Breech Trial
(Hannah et al 2000). Although the findings of this trial have been
disputed (Anonymous 2000) they remain authoritative, and it is
anticipated that one consequence of the study will be a severe
diminution in the clinical skills associated with a normal breech
birth.

The circular effect of changing obstetric practices on the accepted
limits of normality, and on the interventions caused by that diagnosis, can also be explored in the context of length of labour. This
parameter is relevant to all labouring women and their attending
midwives. The 1970 British Births Survey (Chamberlain et al 1978)
proposed an intrapartum scoring system, which scores length of
labour as shown in Table 5.2.

This system is justified by the following statement:

> Duration of first stage of labour—any factor which unduly prolongs
> labour may constitute a risk of intrauterine hypoxia and infection;
> labour has been rated as normal up to 12 hours, as of intermediate
> risk of 12–24 hours, and as a serious problem when extended
> beyond 24 hours. (Chamberlain et al 1978 p 53–54)

It is interesting to ask how this rating system is justified. Since
length of labour is a factor midwives often have to use in judging
the normality or otherwise of labour, it is worth exploring in some
depth.

Berkley et al (1931) suggested that '[l]abour in primiparae lasts
on average about 15 to 20 hours. In multiparae, eight to ten hours
can be taken as the average time. ... It is foolish to attempt to proph-
esy more than approximately how long labour will last in any given
case' (p 273). By 1958 Myles appears to be rather more certain and

her statement uses the language of normality as well as that of the average:

> Seldom is the second stage less than an hour in a primipara and midwives are usually advised to consider 2 hours as being sufficiently long: the multiparous woman may have a second stage of 15 minutes or less and one hour is advocated as the limit of normal. The duration of the third stage is between 10 and 20 minutes, and one hour is recommended as the limit of what could be considered normal. The consensus of opinion is that during the past twenty years the duration of labour has been shorter than previously, probably due to the greater use of relaxation and sedation. The figures below could be considered fairly average but experience proves that average figures can be misleading.

	First stage	Second stage	Third stage	Total
Primigravida	12½	2	½	15
Multipara	8½	1	½	10

> A considerable number of primiparae have labours of under 12 hours, and by far the greater numbers of multiparae have labours of 6 to 8 hours and in many cases less than 6 hours. (Myles 1958 p 228)

Although the possibility of variation is accepted in the text, the only examples given were where labours were shorter than expected. This emphasis is reinforced in a subsequent textbook (Myles 1975 p 211):

	First stage	Second stage	Third stage	Total
Primigravida	11	¾	¼	12
Multipara	6½	½	¼	7

This later edition of Myles' text also stated that the duration of labour had decreased in the last 20 years and added oxytocin to the list of elements considered to have contributed to the change. More recent work by Albers (1999) has indicated that, left to their own devices, a certain percentage of women will labour for up to twice as long as is deemed normal, with no ill effects for themselves or their babies. However, in most acute hospitals it is now almost impossible to ascertain the true limits of normally progressing labour because assumptions of risk associated with long labour have changed obstetric and midwifery practice to the point where labour has been redefined into preset time scales.

It can be argued that one of the factors influencing the change in perception of midwives about the sphere of their practice is that of midwifery regulation and the consequent restriction of midwifery to an increasingly narrowly defined scope of practice. In pursuing this theory, it is of interest to note the historical arguments against the regulation of midwifery. As Donnison (1988) points out, many midwives practising prior to the 1902 Act were against legalisation, feeling that it would bring them under the domination of the medical profession. This view was still current until at least the late 1980s. Mason (1988) describing the debate about the legalisation of midwifery in Canada, comments on the opposition of some lay midwives to the change, on the grounds that it would restrict midwifery. She states that 'pressure mounted on the new almost-legal midwives not to deviate from fairly conservative standards of safe practice at home births.' (Mason 1988 p 125)

The counter argument, now as in 1902, rests on the need for legislation to ensure the maintenance of optimum practice or, more precisely, to allow for the censorship (and deregistration) of bad practitioners. This combination of push and resistance led to the creation of legislation that was based on restriction rather than being enabling. The Midwives Act 1902 in the UK was 'an act to secure the better training of midwives, and to regulate their practice'. There is very little in the Act about training and a lot about regulation, including the setting up of the local supervision authority to 'investigate charges of malpractice, negligence, or misconduct' (Section 8 (2)). The notion of supervision implies that a line between a good and a bad practitioner will have to be drawn. This entails establishing the parameters of safe practice. If there were good and consistent research defining such limits, and the negative outcomes that would result from transcending them, legalisation describing them would be empowering for every midwife. However, this is still not the case, and the regulation of midwifery, of necessity, limits some positive innovative practices in the process of restricting those that may be potentially harmful.

When the 1902 Act was formulated, the concept of normality was not embedded within it. The Act did not mention the limits of midwifery practice or the appropriate time for referral. These were, however, outlined in detail in the 1903 rules (Towler & Bramall 1986 p 181). Although the rules no longer specify in detail what is to be regarded as abnormal, and therefore within the province of the doctor, lack of agreement remains between professions about where the line should be drawn between the normal and the abnormal and who should define that line. This is also an issue within midwifery itself. A study carried out by Oakley & Houd (1990) illustrates the point. The work included an examination of the nature of mid-wifery via interviews with 26 midwives and 21 obstetricians in a number of different European countries. The participants were given specific case histories and asked for their opinion on what they would do in the circumstances (see Tables 5.3 and 5.4).

These tables are of interest, because they reveal that there are not only differences between professionals in different countries but differences between professionals in the same country. However, what is most striking is the expectation of normality or of abnormal outcomes depending on the philosophy of the professionals in each case.

For example, the first UK midwife in Table 5.3 does not expect infection and so does not intervene. However, the Italian obstetrician in the same case is certain that infection will ensue and aggressively manages the case based on that expectation. In Table 5.4, the second Italian obstetrician is adamant that there is a risk of stillbirth and this is uppermost in the decision to induce. The UK midwife, however, while recognising that others would act differently, does not judge the situation to be abnormal and thus does not actively intervene. These case histories indicate the different rules of abnormality operating for different practitioners, and their actions consequent on these rules—even though the case history is the same.

In a recent study commissioned by the Ontario Women's Health Council, researchers examined the characteristics of four Canadian units with low rates of caesarean section (Ontario Women's Health Council 2001). This is in contrast to most work in this area, which has focused on the inexorable rise in rates of caesarean section. The group found that the following 12 characteristics were a feature of these units:

- pride in low C/S rate
- philosophy of birth as a normal physiological process
- commitment to 1–1 support by caregiver during active labour
- strong team leadership
- effective multidisciplinary teams (who liked each other!)
- timely access to skilled professionals
- commitment to evidence-based practice
- programmes to ensure continuous quality improvement
- an accessible and interactive database of outcomes
- continuity and coordination of care both within the hospital and with external services
- well-developed networking
- ability and willingness to manage change.

Table 5.3 Case study: whether or not to intervene (Reproduced with permission from Oakley & Houd 1990 Helpers in Childbirth: Midwifery Today. Hemisphere Publishing Corp, London)

Case	Recommendations from care-givers (summarized)					
	Midwife, United Kingdom	Midwife, Italy	Midwife, United Kingdom	Midwife, Denmark	Obstetrician, Italy	Obstetrician, United Kingdom
A 30-year-old primipara goes into labour a few days past term. Labour starts with ruptured membranes at 6 p.m. At 8 p.m. she is in hospital. She is only dilated about 2 cm. Clear amnion heart beat good. No contractions. What would you do from here?	I wouldn't have her in the hospital anyway. I'd just leave her, I wouldn't do an internal, no nothing. The danger of infection is very little at home anyway. So long as the amnion is clear, I'd let her wait several days	We wait 24 hours, but she must take antibiotics and see the doctor. After that we induce	I'd see if she has had any food, make sure she got her supper, and hope she gets a good night's sleep. If in the morning there hadn't been any action—if we'd done an internal, we would have tried to stir things up a bit—we might even consider an enema. I'd assume she'd want to avoid a drip; well, I would want to avoid a drip. I might encourage her to get up and walk around in the morning. Then after a few hours she'd have to have Syntocinon	I'd ask how she felt—if she was tired or if she was quite fit. I'd give her a massage and see if it caused any contractions. If by midnight she didn't have any, I'd let her sleep. We would have to induce her in the morning	If contractions haven't begun after 6 hours, I'd induce. If the first drip doesn't induce, I'd wait 6 hours and give a second. It's absolutely necessary to give antibiotics, and we must do a culture to make sure there aren't any pathological microbes in the vagina to begin with	I'd probably let her walk around for a while. They have a bath, and if they haven't had their bowels open that day, they get a course of suppositories. You don't normally give enemas, and you don't shave them either. I'd encourage her to walk about, and I'd feed her to give the uterus something to work on, and then I'd just wait and see what happens. If after 12 hours she hadn't done very much, then we'd offer her some Syntocinon. But again if they refuse (they don't usually refuse if you talk to them sensibly), the longer you leave them with the waters gone, the more risk there is to the baby

Table 5.4 Case study: induction (postterm) (Reproduced with permission from Oakley & Houd 1990 *Helpers in Childbirth: Midwifery Today*. Hemisphere Publishing Corp, London)

Case	Obstetrician, Italy	Obstetrician, Italy	Midwife, Greece	Midwife, Italy	Midwife, Denmark	Midwife, United Kingdom
			Recommendations from care-givers (summarized)			
A 28-year-old woman having her second baby is 12 days overdue according to dates and ultrasound. Baby's weight is estimated at 3600 g. Human placental lactogens and oestriol levels are normal. Hormone tests are OK. Her first child weighed 3500 g and was delivered at term +8 days. Her menstrual cycle is 4½–5 weeks. What should be done?	I'd wait until 42 weeks and then I'd do an induction. Meanwhile, I'd give her a kick chart and an amnioscopy every day. I don't take any notice of the menstrual cycle if I have 2 ultrasound scans	I wouldn't have let this pregnancy go over the due date by so many days. We'd have to do a series of tests to be sure the infant is mature first and then induce. After all, we're dealing with a case of potential stillbirth	As a midwife in Greece, I don't have the right to do anything in this case. I'd send the woman to the doctor, and he'll say what has to be done. I wouldn't induce labour. It's up to the doctor	If there's some dilatation of the cervix, I'd suggest an amnioscopy. If the amniotic fluid is clear, I'd wait 2 more days. Then I'd admit her to hospital so as to attempt oxytocic stimulation	First of all, I'd see how she felt psychologically and physically at this stage. Then I'd study her first pregnancy: time of delivery, if she was overdue then, too. Then I'd go back to the ultrasound and do a new calculation, remembering her long cycle. She'd be just about due now. I'd send her to the doctor next time because, according to our directives, she must see the doctor at 41 weeks	I'd check that she is well, still gaining weight, blood pressure normal, etc. I'd suggest that maybe making love might push things on a bit or even a dose of castor oil. She's not too much overdue, and it probably has something to do with her long menstrual cycle. A doctor at this stage would be more inclined to give a date for induction after doing an internal examination, but I'd be inclined to let the mother go longer and encourage the mother to do something herself

This work remains to be tested more widely, and to be measured against the characteristics of units with high rates of caesarean section and other interventions. However, it suggests for the first time that, among other factors, the philosophy of birth prevailing in a maternity setting may have a profound impact on the nature of birth in that setting. This is a revolutionary proposal for a maternity service based on risk and abnormality, and it provides a window of opportunity to enact a paradigm shift in ways of thinking in the future.

CONCLUSION

It is not ground-breaking to make the claim that the definition of the boundaries between normality and abnormality in maternity care is an essential element in understanding the nature of childbirth in any particular society. However, the impact of new technologies on those definitions, and the relative position of power defined by them, is a new phenomenon in the taxonomy of normality and abnormality.

It may well be that the time has come for midwives to begin to recognise that the imposition of an abnormal risk status for women and babies is often not scientific and that while in some cases it promotes benefit, in others it causes iatrogenic damage. Crucially, in many cases it has the consequence that birthing women are divorced from their own experience of birth. If midwives are truly to be the experts in normality, they must also learn to defend definitions of the normal, in order to protect mothers and babies and to promote optimum health gain. The role of lead professional in new forms of maternity care affords an excellent opportunity and a profound challenge to midwifery. For instance, can new technologies be applied sensitively and appropriately by expert midwives to both identify true pathology to empower women in appropriate decision-making, while at the same time preserving the normality of pregnancy and birth? Perhaps more crucially, can midwifery in collaboration with those using the maternity service, bring back a balance between the fear of risk and the belief that birth is usually a positive and life-enhancing process which has no need of technologies? Perhaps the following quotations are the best illustration of where this debate needs to go from here.

> The midwife's clinical knowledge … provides [the mother] with a safe and cherished space in which to cope … Such holding increases

the space in which the mother can act: it does not restrain her …
[but] … very often the clinicians' technical expertise holds clients in
a grip which constrains their freedom of action and inhibits their
instinctive responses. (Walters & Kirkham 1997 p 109)

Each one of us has the continuing and increasing responsibility to
ask the question, 'although we can do this, ought we to do it?'
(James & Stirrat 1988 p 4)

References

Albers L L 1999 The duration of labor in healthy women. Journal of Perinatology
    19:114–119

[Anonymous] 2000 The 'term breech trial': a multicentre study finds caesarean
    section best. International Midwifery 13(6):10

Arney W R 1982 Power and the profession of obstetrics. The University of
    Chicago Press, Chicago

Bennett V R, Brown L K (eds) 1999 Myles textbook for midwives, 13th edn.
    Churchill Livingstone, Edinburgh

Berkeley C et al 1931 Midwifery by ten teachers, 4th edn. Edward Arnold,
    London

Butler N R, Alberman E D, Peel J 1969 Perinatal problems: the second report of
    the 1958 British Perinatal Mortality Survey. E & S Livingstone, Edinburgh

Campbell R 1999 Review and assessment of selection criteria used when booking
    pregnant women at different places of birth. British Journal of Obstetrics &
    Gynaecology 106:550–556

Chamberlain G et al 1978 British births 1970: a survey under the joint auspices of
    the National Birthday Trust Fund and the Royal College of Obstetricians and
    Gynaecologists, volume 2 Obstetric care. Heinemann Medical, London

Daker M, Bobrow M 1989 Screening for genetic disease. In: Enkin M, Keirse M,
    Chalmers I (eds) A guide to effective care in pregnancy and childbirth. Oxford
    University Press, Oxford

Dodd V 1999 Court to decide on HIV test for baby. Parents claim daughter's
    health should be their responsibility. The Guardian Tuesday 24 August

Donnison J 1988 Midwives and medical men: a history of the struggle for the
    control of childbirth. Historical Publications, New Barnet

Downe S M, McCormick C, Beech B 2001 Labour interventions associated with
    normal birth. British Journal of Midwifery 9:602–606

Edge V, Laros R K Jr 1993 Pregnancy outcome in nulliparous women aged 35 and
    older. American Journal of Obstetrics and Gynecology 168:1881–1885

Enkin M et al (eds) 2000 A guide to effective care in pregnancy and childbirth, 3rd
    edn. Oxford University Press, Oxford

Handwerker L 1994 Medical risk: implicating poor pregnant women. Social
    Science and Medicine 3:665–675

Hannah M E, Hannah W J, Hewson S A et al 2000 Planned caesarean section
    versus planned vaginal birth for breech presentation at term: a randomised
    multicentre trial. Term Breech Trial Collaborative Group. Lancet
    356:1375–1383

James D K, Stirrat G M (eds) 1988 Pregnancy and risk: the basis for rational management. John Wiley, Chichester

Leap N, Hunter B 1993 The midwives tale: an oral history from handywomen to professional midwife. Scarlet Press, London

Lilford R J et al 1983 Maternal levels of human placental lactogen in the prediction of fetal growth retardation: choosing a cut-off point between normal and abnormal. British Journal of Obstetrics and Gynaecology 90:511–515

Mason J 1988 Midwifery in Canada. In: Kitzinger S (ed) The midwife challenge. Pandora Press, London

Myles M F 1958 A textbook for midwives, 3rd edn. Livingstone, Edinburgh

Myles M F 1975 A textbook for midwives, 8th edn. Churchill Livingstone, Edinburgh

Oakley A, Houd S 1990 Helpers in childbirth; midwifery today. WHO, Regional Office for Europe, Hemisphere Publishing corporation, London

Ontario Women's Health Council 2001 Attaining and maintaining best practices in the use of caesarean sections. Online. Available: http://www.womenshealthcouncil.com/E/index.html

Rosenthal A N, Paterson-Brown S 1998 Is there an incremental rise in the risk of obstetric intervention with increasing maternal age? British Journal of Obstetrics and Gynaecology 105:1064–1069

Rothman B K 1994 The tentative pregnancy: amniocentesis and the sexual politics of motherhood. Pandora Press, London

Sackett D L 2000 Evidence-based medicine: how to practice and teach EBM. Wolfe, Edinburgh

Thomas J, Paranjothy S 2001 The National Sentinel Caesarean Section Audit Report. Available: Royal College of Obstetrics and Gynaecologists, Clinical Effectiveness Support Unit, RCOG Press, London

Towler J, Bramall J 1986 Midwives in history & society. Croom Helm, Beckenham

Walters D, Kirkham M J 1997 Doulas and midwives. In: Kirkham M J, Perkins E R Reflections on midwifery. Bailliére Tindall, London

Wolf L E, Lo B, Beckerman K P et al 2001 When parents reject interventions to reduce postnatal human immunodeficiency virus transmission. Archives of Pediatrics and Adolescent Medicine 155:927–933

Chapter **6**

Midwives and sexuality: earth mother or coy maiden

Catherine Williams

INTRODUCTION

In this chapter I explore the relationship between sexuality, the reproductive continuum, and the midwife. Initially, various personal experiences will be recounted that led me to suggest that the medicalisation of childbirth has divorced sexuality from childbirth and has created the coy maiden midwife, at the expense of the earth mother midwife. These experiences are from my work as a health care worker in the late 1970s and early 1980s and also, more recently, from my work as a lecturer to student health professionals in higher education.

Having established that there does clearly seem to be a sexual component in the reproductive continuum, I suggest that the writing out or exclusion of sexuality in this context actually complicates, confuses and blurs the issues rather than making the sexual aspect safe. I suggest that all health professionals, particularly midwives, need to recognise and acknowledge the sexual nature of their work in order to be able to relate honestly to and support the person seeking their professional assistance.

PROFESSIONAL EXPERIENCES

Looking back, the initial encounter that led me to question the relationship between sexuality and midwives occurred during a 3-month obstetric course prior to starting my health visiting training. The specific incident was my first vaginal examination (VE). I can remember my response as if it were yesterday—I was stunned by how lovely her vagina was, how soft, warm, velvety and moist. I can remember saying 'Oh isn't it lovely, so warm and soft? Isn't it a nice place to be? No wonder men like sex so much', as I gently explored the woman's vagina and tried to locate what the midwife was describing. The woman whom I was examining seemed to enjoy my enthusiasm and smiled, remaining relaxed. The midwife suggested that I should remove my fingers and that was enough. Nothing was said, but I was aware that I had transgressed one of those invisible rules that one meets occasionally in life. To put this in context, it was in the mid-1970s, women's consciousness raising had not happened yet in the North West of England, or if it had it had certainly passed me by. The National Childbirth Trust movement was around but very much a fringe activity and was disapproved of by most of the midwives I came across. At that time I was not sure what rule I had transgressed, but now I realise. To link the clinical VE with sex was a major sin. Not only that, but actually enjoying it and expressing my enjoyment of another woman's body was clearly a mortal sin in the midwifery world. Childbirth was clearly divorced from sexuality, it was a medical not a sexual event.

Since then, having worked as a health visitor and then training and working as a midwife, I have never, in the professional context, heard anyone mention how lovely a woman's vagina is or the possibility of a VE being enjoyable in any way. The emphasis has always been placed on the diagnostic function, one that is acknowledged to be very intrusive, may be uncomfortable and painful for the woman and rightly kept to the minimum in terms of frequency and duration. Recent discussion is even questioning its value both antenatally, during labour and postnatally (Clement 1994). Here I feel the need to make it clear that I was not getting a sexual buzz out of the situation but that I was acknowledging and enjoying the woman as a sexual being in the very sexual act of childbirth. It was very similar to the enjoyment and wonder I felt every time I was present at the spiritual and sexual moment of birth. Looking back at my midwifery experiences I see that I learnt very quickly not to express or acknowledge the sexual aspect of childbirth at all.

The sacred or spiritual was a permissible outlet at times in response to particular women and their babies, but mostly it was overridden by the medicalisation of the whole event; everything was transformed into the clinical. Clinical with a humane side certainly, clinical with a natural aspect too, but working in an NHS hospital this clinical perspective dominated.

I had always expected that midwives would be the ultimate earth mother, a grounded sensual, sexy woman who was in touch with the rhythms of the seasons. To be socialised into a medicalised coy maiden midwife had been a real challenge to my assumptions. I would like to suggest a midwifery continuum with two images of the midwife at either end. At one end we have the earth mother, the grounded, raunchy home-birthing midwife, who perceives childbirth not only as a life event but also as a sensual and sacred event. At this end of the midwifery continuum we have Gaskin (1980) saying '[e]very birth is holy I think that a midwife must be religious, because the energy she is dealing with is Holy. She needs to know that other people's energy is sacred.'

Gaskin goes on to explain that by religion she means that 'compassion must be a way of life' for the midwife. Another view of what I shall call the earth mother midwife is from Kitzinger (1991) who cites the Tao Te Ching's description:

> You are a midwife: you are assisting at someone else's birth. Do good without show or fuss. Facilitate what is happening rather than lead what you think ought to be happening. If you must take the lead, lead so that the mother is helped, yet still free and in charge. When the baby is born, the mother will rightly say: 'We did it ourselves'.

This earth mother midwife is 100% there for the birthing woman, endlessly giving, intuitive, sensitive, open, accepting, compassionate, loving, meeting her every need, truly holistic. A very wise woman.

At the other end of the continuum we have the medicalised midwife—the coy maiden—standing behind or beside the rest of the professional team within the masculine patriarchal obstetric system. Kitzinger (1991) starts one of her books: 'In child birth today the obstetrician usually stands centre-stage. The midwife is invisible.'

This midwife may also be endlessly giving, kind, sensitive and aiming to meet the needs of the birthing woman but she is also a product of her culture, the medical culture. She is endlessly connecting up the tubes and wires of technology and meeting the needs of the medical model. Not only has she (in England, at present) most probably been socialised into the nursing role, and all that entails, prior to becoming a midwife, but most of her midwifery socialisation will be well within the medical model and she will be very fortunate if she has ever been present at a home birth.

I am not putting this midwife down, she may be, and probably is, a wonderful woman, but to stay in-touch with the social, sexual and sacred aspects of childbirth in the sterile, aseptic, technical world of obstetrics is very hard. The midwives stand in coy uniforms that are reminiscent of the serving class, trying to meet the needs of very different groups of people—the pregnant women, the obstetrician's team and the hospital management structure. In these circumstances it is very difficult to become grounded enough to start to fight for the woman's needs. And a fight is not a good starting point for her to reach her goal of being 'with' the birthing woman.

Most midwives in this country are probably somewhere along the continuum placed between the two extremes. My fear is that most are clustered towards the coy maiden end.

Three recent incidents, in particular, have led me to analyse further the relationship between midwives, childbirth and sexuality and I intend to outline them briefly prior to developing my discussion.

The first was during a fairly informal interprofessional meeting. We broke for coffee and I realised that I had started bleeding early and had no sanitary wear. I came back into the group and stated that I had started bleeding and asked if anyone had any tampons I could use. One of the midwives said 'Oh yes' and disappeared out of the room. A few minutes later she came back in and came up to me and whispered that she had put 'what I needed on top of the loo'. I felt I had been 'coy maiden midwifed'. I value the care, the concern and the thoughtfulness of her discretion, but it highlighted to me the 'coy maiden' approach to midwifery where discretion *can* become a barrier to naming what is, so concealing and silencing the reality and sexuality of women's reproduction. My bleeding is about being a woman, it is about my reproductive potential and it is about my sexuality. I do not want it concealed and made invisible as it so often is in our patriarchal society. This is often what we do to women who we meet in our jobs as midwives: we sanitise it, we create a discreet clinical barrier between us and most aspects of the reproductive continuum, from menstruation, through contraception, conception, assisted conception, antenatal interactions, childbirth and the postnatal period. This may well suit a lot of women who also view the process in a clinical way, but where is the sexual and the sacred for the women who do want to express their reproductive lives in this other way?

The second incident occurred while I was teaching about sexuality on the Midwifery Diploma course. The students were mature and qualified nurses. We did an exercise that focused on their own bodies and their own sexuality. There was a lot of resistance and reluctance to address the issue of their own sexuality. It was more acceptable to address the sexuality of the 'other', the patient, and work with that but not to address their own. I also find this tendency with some of the student nurses I teach. In contrast, some other groups of students I teach and do the same exercise with, who have nothing to do with health professions, express much less resistance and engage in it enthusiastically. Interestingly during the lunch break after the exercise the student midwives started talking informally and when I returned they were wild. Barriers had dropped and the conversation was more like the end of a 'girls' night out' and the level of bawdiness made Chaucer's *Canterbury Tales* seem polite! It reminded me of coffee break talk on the labour ward, especially on late or night shift. As one colleague said to me 'get a group of midwives together and it's all orgasms and penises'. So here we seem to have the 'coy maiden' operating in the formal context but in the informal context we perhaps see aspects of the 'earth mother'. Is it that the medicalised midwife is so repressed in the 'coy maiden' role but so much in constant touch with bodies and raw sexuality in her everyday work, that she needs some outlet and once this is provided, out it pours? Would it not be better for sexuality to be an acknowledged part of the midwife–client relationship?

The third incident again involves my teaching role and my increasing awareness of the complications in the lives of the students. When I teach subjects such as domestic and sexual violence, the number of students who have experienced abuse is significant. This undoubtedly reflects the increasing awareness and incidence of child sexual abuse and rape in our society at large (Scully 1990, Tidy 1994), so is not surprising in itself. However, it does have implications for the health professions, particularly midwifery, because the focus is on the sexual event of reproduction. Certain sessions have aroused deep pain for some of the women students and I feel particular concern about whether they can help others if they are not healed themselves.

So where does sexuality come into all this? The two main discourses Cosslett (1994) has identified—the 'natural' and 'the medical'—will be employed to look at what role sexuality plays. I will then discuss what the implications are for the midwife and the midwife–client relationship if we do not acknowledge the reproductive continuum as a sexual process.

WHERE DOES SEXUALITY COME INTO ALL THIS?

Birth is the biological end result of heterosexual intercourse, on the occasions that conception takes place, so on this biological level we can fairly assuredly assert that childbirth is a sexual event. However, with the increasing development of contraception, the gap between heterosexual intercourse and conception has been steadily widening. Add to this the developments in assisted conception and the two become even further apart; conception itself becomes a clinical event and sometimes even a scientific laboratory event.

Cosslett (1994) suggests that there are three discourses of motherhood: the natural, the medical and the old wives' tales. The two images of the midwife that I am using in this chapter, the coy handmaiden and the earth mother, neatly fit into two of the main discourses.

Additionally, sexuality is more than heterosexual intercourse, though this is sometimes difficult to perceive in late 20th-century English culture and, rather than get into a long discussion on the cultural construction of sexuality, I would simply like to quote from the book *Our Bodies Ourselves*:

> Sexuality is much more than intercourse. It is a pleasure we want to give and receive. It is a vital expression of attachment to other human beings. It is communication that is fun, playful, serious and passionate ... sexual feelings and responses are a central expression of our emotional, spiritual, physical selves. Sexual feelings involve our whole bodies. (Phillips & Rakusen 1979 p 30–31)

Natural childbirth discourse and the earth mother midwife

In England Kitzinger is probably the most well known natural childbirth proponent and educator. She argues that childbirth is 'part of a woman's whole psychosexual life—not simply ... an isolated occurrence at one end of her body' (1979 p 11).

Some of the women from the 'Farm Community in Tennessee' write about their experiences in Gaskin's book *Spiritual Midwifery* (Gaskin 1980). I quote some of them to illustrate the sexual nature of their experience of childbirth. 'The rushes [contractions] started to turn me on. It feels like William [her partner] and I learned how to kiss each other in a heavier way than we'd been into before' (1980 p 42).

Karen also talked of her labour in similar vein:

> My rushes hardly felt heavy at all, but I knew they must be because I was opening up. We just kept making out and rubbing each other.

We got to places that we had forgotten we could get to. Since that day we have been remembering to really get it on. Going through the birthing I felt his love very strong. It was like getting married all over again. (1980 p 43)

Another woman, Cara, who trained to be a midwife at the Farm says: 'Over and over again I've seen the best way to get a baby out is by cuddling and smooching with your husband. That loving sexy vibe is what puts the baby in there and it's what gets it out, too' (Gaskin 1980 p 52).

Rabuzzi (1994) suggests there is a growing body of accounts of childbirth that not only acknowledge, but celebrate, the sexual aspect. She cites Moran's research into home birthing to give another insight into the erotic aspect of childbirth.

I dreamt of John holding me tenderly during labour and after the baby was born—like RIGHT after. Naturally this happened! It was a natural response to the love and the sexual aspect of birth. (Rabuzzi 1994 p 120)

A husband of another woman having a home birth said:

The birth was not only painless, but very pleasurable. We had never read about this aspect, and it took us both by surprise. As the baby crowned, I knew from Jean's look and sounds that she was having an explosive orgasm, which rolled on and on. What a long way from the pain and agony of conventional myth. (Rabuzzi 1994 p 120)

So there is clearly much evidence from heterosexual women, their partners and their midwives in the natural birth movement to support the suggestion that childbirth is a sexual event.

Likewise women have described pregnancy as being a very sexual and erotic time for them. Chesler (cited in Rabuzzi 1994), addresses her unborn child:

I want to have orgasms without foreplay three or four times every day. I look at your father slyly, passively. I insist he come back to bed, 'now'. If we're outside, I suggest we borrow a friend's bedroom, or sneak into a hotel restroom, just for a minute.

I am without shame. Never have I been in such sexual heat. Is this natural in pregnancy? Or am I enjoying my lust because I think it unnatural, taboo? What exactly is so arousing, so pleasurably 'lewd' to me about a woman with a round, fat belly initiating orgasms in Mediterranean heat? Is my body remembering something? Can bodies do this? ... During and after love-making I watch my stomach, I watch you, like a voyeur, as if I'm not present. There's a direct line from my *consciousness* of your existence to my clitoris. Watching my belly, having my belly seen by another, seems to throb this mysterious line awake.

My serpent rises lazily, a full four feet, then coils back into its clitoral hood. My tiger is gone, my tiger returns, restless, ready to prowl again. (1994 p 119)

This delicious quote says it all and contrasts strongly with my experience as a midwife in the medical model when pregnant women frequently asked whether it was all right to have sexual intercourse with their partner and whether it would harm the baby. It was as though they had lost their power to decide and feel what was right for themselves.

Rabuzzi (1994) also suggests the possibility of an erotic relationship between the woman and the fetus. They are united as one and once the woman actually feels movements she can feel another being inside her and as Rabuzzi says this, 'opens up a whole new dimension of sexual experience'. She questions whether there is a closer relationship and suggests that from quickening to birth, 'the two relate as romance promises all lovers do. This is the bliss every lover craves.'

Clearly natural childbirth has a lot to say about the sexual experience of pregnancy and childbirth and there is also much evidence (Gaskin 1980, Rabuzzi 1994, Stanway & Stanway 1978) to support the connection between sexuality and breastfeeding. The midwife clearly needs to be an 'earth mother' to facilitate these women's experiences.

Medical discourse and the coy maiden midwife

In great contrast to the natural childbirth discourse medical discourse, Cosslett (1994) suggests, is that of male technological and scientific procedures taking childbirth out of the hands of women and setting it in the context of the powerful, male-dominated institution of the hospital. The natural childbirth context, however, seemed to be focused very much on the home birth and the power of the woman.

So where does sexuality fit in the context of pregnancy and childbirth in the medical environment? Rabuzzi cites a male obstetrician's observations:

For years, convinced of the fact that delivery of the head constituted, owing to the perineal distension, the most painful phase of childbirth, we traditionally administered an anaesthetic to the parturient. It is striking to observe that women who have been conditioned by the psychoprophylactic method frequently declare that delivery of the head affords them the most exhilarating moment of the entire event. Indeed, we have frequently observed that the birth of the head, far from producing the usual tearing pain, stimulates an intense thrill, very close to that of orgasm. (1994 p 103)

It is interesting that he links the sexual experience of childbirth to women who have trained in psychoprophylaxis and are therefore likely to have links with the natural childbirth movement. Rabuzzi clearly sees this obstetrician as an exception and suggests that patriarchal culture has such a block against seeing any potential for the erotic in childbirth that all the sensations are conventionally labelled pain or discomfort.

I remember while working on a postnatal ward a woman asked me for an early discharge. Her answer to my enquiry as to the reason was that she felt so sexual after the whole experience of childbirth and breastfeeding that she wanted to get back to her partner as quickly as possible. Clearly, some women can find the experience sexual in the medical setting.

However, as many of us know, sexuality is not all bliss, orgasms and the earth moving. It can also be about miscommunication, misinterpretation, pressure, powerlessness, feeling empty, fear, failure, abuse and violence to name a few. Kitzinger (1992) has written about how for many women childbirth can become an 'ordeal in which they are disempowered' (p 68). She compares the language these women use to describe childbirth to the language used when describing experiences of sexual violence. Kitzinger clearly points out that this is not an experience only to be found in hospital; women were also writing of horrific experiences of childbirth at home 40 years ago. But with the increase in technology, intervention and a medicalised and hospitalised childbirth the opportunity for intervention has increased. Many of the women writing to Kitzinger had been subjected to a technological childbirth and they used words such as 'rape', 'assault', 'abuse' and 'violence' in the description of their childbirth experience. Kitzinger (1992) suggests that the theme of powerlessness is common to the women and goes on to show the clear similarities between powerless childbirth and rape; from the physical pain and damage, the lack of personal identity, to the emotional blackmail that can be used to ensure the patient or victim goes along with it. 'In childbirth, as in rape, a woman may be stripped, forcibly exposed, her legs splayed and tethered and her sexual organs put on display to all comers' (p 73).

She goes on to say that when women describe it they use the 'language of pornography' (Kitzinger 1992 p 74). The women often blame themselves, and again, as in rape, the professionals involved often reinforce this. Kitzinger clearly shows the similarities of the women who feel they have been violated by the obstetric management of their labour and women who have been raped. The connection between childbirth and sexuality is all too clear in her analysis of these women's accounts. She concludes: 'Rape is endemic in our society. The western way of birth proves often to be another form of institutionalised violence against women' (p 78).

SO WHERE IS THE EARTH MOTHER AND THE COY MAIDEN?

Indeed where is the midwife in all this? In Kitzinger's (1992) chapter discussed above there is only occasional mention of the midwife. She focuses on technological intervention and male violence at an institutional level as an explanation. Rabuzzi, from the USA, focuses on the male patriarchal obstetrician when considering the medical model. When discussing what she calls the 'midwifery model' she focuses very much on midwives like Gaskin whose emphasis is on a spiritual and community experience in the home environment—very much the earth mother image of the midwife. In fact the midwife gets off very lightly in many current critiques of the process of childbearing. I wonder if this is justified. Where are the midwives during these labours where women feel abused and raped? Are they coy maidens standing by the side of the woman, being 'with' the woman but also being endlessly discreet and caring, not seeing the situation as abusive because it is shrouded in the clinical medical terminology of 'being in the patient's interests'? Are they so co-opted into the male medical system that they see the situation through the male medical gaze rather than from a gynocentric view? Do they not see it because childbirth is a medical event and not a sexual event? If they perceived the whole process as a sexual event that is important in women's lives would that change things? Could it alter their perception?

O'Driscoll (1994) has presented some brief case studies, one was of a woman who refused to be examined by the doctor antenatally. It was the midwife who explained the reasons for the examination and despite the woman's fear it was done. The woman had been gang-raped as a teenager and could not tell the midwife as 'she [the midwife] was very busy' (p 39). O'Driscoll states that '[s]ometimes the midwife is a prime player but not always to good effect' (p 39). I think it is important to recognise the midwives' role in these situations—they must not be the doctors' handmaidens standing on the side lines, reinforcing the status quo.

Tidy (1994) also graphically illustrates in her case study how going through childbirth can bring back hidden memories of child abuse. I quote at length as this woman's experience makes such a clear point:

> … she coped well throughout the first stage, but the change to the second stage caused her to panic as she felt the baby descend through her pelvis. The similarity between an adult penis being forced inside the body of an 8-year-old and a fetus descending through the birth canal must be striking. When she shouted for help, the midwife used the exact words her abuser had used, 'Shh—don't cry!' reinforcing her feeling of abuse. (p 388–389)

O'Driscoll (1994) sympathetically discusses the role of midwives in relation to childbirth and sexuality, suggesting that they need to, 'explore their own reactions' to vaginal examinations and that they need to 'remember that touch, pain and physical examinations can unlock hidden terrors' (p 40). She suggests a feminist approach, encouraging a midwife to be assertive and to act as an advocate for the woman. This is moving from coy maiden midwife further down the midwifery continuum towards the earth mother.

I would go further and suggest that not only do midwives need to look at their own feelings about vaginal examinations but they need to thoroughly explore their own issues around sexuality and then apply this understanding to the process and interactions around childbearing in our culture. I suggest that all midwifery education, especially refresher courses, should have space for initiating and developing this sexual awareness of midwives. Hopefully this in turn will enable them in Kitzinger's (1993) words to 'ensure that the care they offer counteracts rather than re-enacts the violation of women's bodies' (p 220).

The coy maiden midwife often appears to me to be without awareness of her sexuality. Yes, she may be very 'sexy' as male defined, but she has not got in touch with her own female definition of what is sexual. I think this is socialised out of the midwife during both her nurse and midwifery education. Sexuality, although now much discussed and talked about, is somehow paradoxically still a very private area full of taboos.

In the medical model sexuality is mostly medicalised in order, perhaps, to control it and make it safe. Modern obstetric relations reproduce the perceived heterosexual norm of our society. The male obstetrician is in charge of and in control of women's bodies and the women on the whole comply. With this clinical attitude and environment, discretion and professional distancing put up barriers to the dangerous sexual element and hence this is controlled and made safe.

But safe for whom? Certainly not safe for the women who write about their experiences to Kitzinger in terms of 'rape', 'violence' and 'abuse', nor the others that seek or do not seek help for the problems following childbirth that O'Driscoll has highlighted. Is the medicalisation of childbirth actually trying to create safety from women's sexuality and the sacred power of women's creativity? Rabuzzi (1994) explores how through mythology the sacred act of creativity has been taken from women and given to men. She suggests that since men do not have this natural means of connecting to the sacred, they need to create it in their culture and diminish women's natural connection to the sacred through controlling childbirth. Is today's obstetrician the modern-day equivalent of Zeus giving birth to Dionysus? In a patriarchal society the male needs to be in control, have power over, and even more importantly, have a role in reproduction and creativity.

Perhaps the male medicalisation of reproduction also controls women's sexual relations around childbirth by reasserting the heterosexual norm of male power and control. In a more gynocentric approach to childbirth, where the sexual and sacred element of childbirth was recognised as part of the process, the relationship between the birthing woman and the midwife could be a lot more intimate and intense. Rabuzzi (1994), discussing a midwifery model of labour and delivery, points out that these midwives see their role as a holistic process:

> A key word in this process is community—the community to which the childbearing woman belongs and the community that the midwife creates with her, for the relationship that develops between a labouring woman and her birth attendant is often astonishingly close … it can also create community at a very deep level. (p 86)

She reinforces this picture by quoting O'Dent's observations of the midwife at work: 'Body to body, skin to skin, a midwife will rely on touching and holding a woman, rather than speaking to her' (p 86).

Both O'Dent and Rabuzzi talk of the relationship as 'communion'. 'Communion at its holiest, this sharing of the creating of new life clearly manifests the sacred dimension of childbearing' (Rabuzzi 1994 p 86). It also clearly demonstrates the sexual dimension of the relationship. This intimate intense woman-to-woman relationship clearly challenges the perceived norm of heterosexuality. Perhaps homophobia and in particular the fear of women's close relationships is another factor behind the male medicalisation of reproduction and the creation of barriers between professional and patient. If the midwife has not explored her own attitudes, ideas, assumptions and prejudices around sexuality this may seriously affect her interaction and relationships in her occupation. She may assume the woman is heterosexual, which may lead her to give inappropriate advice, for instance, suggest contraception or ask inappropriate questions about the father of the baby. Presumption of a heterosexual lifestyle can lead the woman to feel very undermined (Rose & Platzer 1993). With lesbophobia so common in nursing (Eliason & Randall 1991) we may presume it to be similar in midwifery. Tash & Kenney (1993) cite an American study where lesbians described, 'ostracism, invasive personal questions, shock, embarrassment, unfriendliness, pity, condescension and fear from health caregivers' (p 37). Not exactly 'the body to body, skin to skin' experience that I cited earlier. Lesbophobia may cause the midwife to withdraw from this intimate intense woman-to-woman relationship.

THE WOUNDED HEALER

If we add to this quagmire of complex human relationships the midwives I mentioned earlier, those who are themselves victims of child and adult sexual abuse, the situation becomes even more difficult. If the midwife herself has been abused and has not worked it through and is with a woman in labour who is going through an experience which she describes later as, 'I feel invaded and mutilated … I don't feel the same person any more' (Kitzinger 1992 p 72), it is no wonder that she cannot speak up, cannot defend the woman and cannot be the woman's advocate.

I return to my point about midwifery education and the essential inclusion of sexuality within preregistration and postregistration courses. I would also recommend this area of education for *all* other health professional education (and I include doctors under this heading) but argue that for midwives it is even more important due to the sexual and intimate nature of their work. It is important for the woman who has been sexually abused to work through her experience, come to some understanding of it and, with help, lay some of the trauma to one side so that she can be more comfortable with her own sexuality and thereby, hopefully, be more comfortable with other people's when she is working in a healing capacity. It is very difficult to heal someone else's wound when one's own wounds are bleeding profoundly and are intensely painful. We need to heal our own wounds before we attempt to heal others.

CONCLUSION

Woman's sexuality represents the interface between two of the most potent and insidious forms of oppression—gender and sexuality. (Gordon & Kanstrup 1992 p 29)

We need to move the pregnant woman centre stage, closely accompanied by the midwife, and diminish the power and influence of the medical model and the obstetrician. The woman-centred care advocated in *Changing Childbirth* (Department of Health 1993) sets the scene for this to happen. This, combined with recent changes in midwifery education such as increasing the numbers of centres that now provide direct entry to midwifery and more midwives moving into higher education, opens doors to change. Through education midwives can be taught to examine and challenge the status quo. They can be encouraged to address the issues of sexuality and move away from the coy maiden towards the earth mother. Not in any way to impose this on women, the last thing we want is for the pregnant woman to feel that she 'ought' to experience it sexually as some women do in natural childbirth. But we need to recognise the diversity of women's needs and the complexity of the sexual aspect of the reproductive continuum in order to enable women to do what they need to do and midwives to support them in whatever choices they make. So to paraphrase the O'Driscoll (1994) quote I used earlier, we need the midwife to be the prime player in the professional team but *always* to *good* effect. Thus it becomes an ethical imperative to make sure that midwifery practice is guided by the principle of beneficence and what the exercising of this principle means in practice must be based on a deeper understanding of women's experiences of childbirth.

Ignoring sexuality or allowing it to be subsumed under the medical model into a clinical event rather than a sexual life event is rather like trying to plug a volcano with liquid cement. We will all get splattered eventually. We need to acknowledge that a sexual relationship is present in our professional relationships. Failure to recognise this as midwives means that we restrict women's needs for both sexual privacy and sexual expression.

References

Clement S 1994 Unwanted vaginal examinations. British Journal of Midwifery 2:368–370

Cosslett T 1994 Women writing childbirth: modern discourses of motherhood. Manchester University Press, Manchester

Department of Health 1993 Changing childbirth. HMSO, London

Eliason M J, Randall C E 1991 Lesbian phobia in nursing students. Western Journal of Nursing Research 13:363–374

Gaskin I M 1980 Spiritual midwifery. The Book Publishing Co, Summertown

Gordon G, Kanstrup C 1992 Sexuality—the missing link in women's health. Ids Bulletin 23:29–37

Kitzinger J 1993 Counteracting, not re-enacting, the violation of women's bodies: the challenge for perinatal caregivers. Birth 19:219–220

Kitzinger S 1979 Education and counselling for childbirth. Schocken Books, New York

Kitzinger S 1991 The midwife challenge. Pandora, London

Kitzinger S 1992 Birth and violence against women. Generating hypotheses from women's accounts of unhappiness after childbirth. In: Roberts H (ed) Women's health matters. Routledge, London, p 63–80

O'Driscoll M 1994 Midwives, childbirth and sexuality. British Journal of Midwifery 2:39–41

Phillips A, Rakusen J 1979 Our bodies ourselves. Penguin, Middlesex

Rabuzzi K A 1994 Mother with child. Indiana University Press, Bloomington

Rose P, Platzer H 1993 Confronting prejudice. Nursing Times 89:52–54

Scully D 1990 Understanding sexual violence. Unwin Hyman, Boston

Stanway P, Stanway A 1978 Breast is best. Pan, London

Tash D T, Kenney J W 1993 The lesbian childbearing couple: a case report. Birth 20:36–40

Tidy H 1994 Effects of child sexual abuse on the experience of childbirth. British Journal of Midwifery 2:387–389

PART 2

Technological issues

Chapter 7

Ethical issues in neonatal intensive care

Pam Miller

INTRODUCTION

Few people with any interest in the subject can be unaware of the immense changes that have taken place in neonatal intensive care over the last few years. Treatment is offered to ever smaller and more immature babies, equipment for measuring every conceivable parameter is constantly refined and most vital functions can now be sustained, for some time at least, by some form of machinery.

It has, however, been said that 'the machinery in an intensive care unit is more sophisticated than the codes of law and ethics governing its use' (Lee & Morgan 1989 p 211). Those who work in neonatal intensive care units usually do so because they enjoy combining the care of babies with developing technological skills. These skills have to be augmented by an understanding of the ethical questions that might arise in this environment. This chapter will attempt to consider some of the ethical issues that confront nurses and midwives working in neonatal intensive care units, addressing such questions as: should all babies born alive be offered intensive care regardless of gestation? What should be the criteria for withdrawing intensive care? How should dying babies and those born with genetic abnormalities be managed? And finally, how should scarce resources best be used?

APPROACHES TO DECISION-MAKING

Initially it may be helpful to look at some of the beliefs that influence decision-makers in the neonatal field. Walters (1988) described four recognised decision-making approaches and it is likely that those involved in making ethical decisions base them on one or more of these positions, even if they could not define it so exactly. Walters' four approaches are as follows:

1. Value of life: this is the principle that every life is sacred and that factors such as quality of life and the cost of treatment have no bearing. This principle is most strongly developed in the Judaeo-Christian belief that man is created in the image of God, but it is also affirmed by most other major world religions (Whyte 1989). One of the possible consequences of denying this principle was seen in the philosophy of the Nazi party in the 1930s where some lives were deemed 'not worthy to be lived' (Ramsey 1982 p xv). Ignoring the intrinsic value of human life may also undermine the public's faith in the medical profession. However, most of those who adhere to this belief also include quality of life considerations when making decisions about a baby's treatment.

2. Parental authority: this approach sees the parents as the rightful decision-makers for infants who are unable to make their own decisions. Since parents are responsible for most of the decisions about their children's upbringing while they are minors, it is inconsistent to deny them this right in the neonatal period. They will also have to bear the brunt of the care of any child who is impaired. However, during the emotionally fraught time after the birth of a very immature or abnormal baby the parents may not be in a fit state to make crucial decisions, nor may they necessarily be able to grasp the degree of impairment anticipated and what that might mean for their child. It is also debatable whether a parent should feel that the responsibility for their child's life or death rests solely with them, although many parents do see this responsibility as the logical sequel to having conceived the child (McHaffie 2001).

3. Best interests: here the baby's best interests are seen as the criteria on which to base decision-making, and treatment should
result in a net benefit to the infant. Although a high value is
placed on the infant's life, this approach recognises that aggres-
sive intervention will not always be in the child's perceived best
interests. However, this approach, although basically rooted in
common sense, is of limited use because it is difficult for anyone
to be certain what the baby's best interests are, both because the
prognosis is often uncertain and because no one can know what
the infant would choose, if in a position to do so.

4. Personhood: in direct contrast to the belief in the sanctity of life,
this concept claims that only the possession of certain capabilities such as self-consciousness, the ability to reason and a sense
of the future confer personhood, and therefore the right to life.
As neither the fetus nor the neonate possess these capabilities
they are not persons and therefore have no automatic right to
life. Proponents of this view, for example Kuhse & Singer (1985),
qualify their position by reasoning that even though neonates
have no intrinsic right to life, if wanted by their parents or by
adoptive parents, it would be wronging them to kill them. Wyatt
(1998) points out that the philosophy of Kuhse & Singer is far
removed from the intuitions of most ordinary people, and Walters
(1988) himself cannot see this approach gaining much credence
among staff and parents in neonatal units in countries with a
basically Christian heritage such as Britain.

Walters (1988) acknowledges that all these approaches are in some
way unsatisfactory in providing a formula for settling hard questions
and goes on to suggest a further approach, which he calls 'proximate
personhood'. The central contention of this approach is that all newborns whose lives approximate personhood should receive at least
ordinary treatment. Approximation to personhood concerns the state
of the child at birth and the potential for development. If a normal
newborn baby, or a baby with minor abnormalities, has reasonable
potential to develop the capabilities of personhood, appropriate treatment should be administered. Walters sees the paediatrician as the
person best qualified to determine the baby's potential and plan
appropriate treatment in consultation with the parents. Since this
approach does not deny the basic right to life, it has something to
offer those who cannot accept the extreme personhood argument.

Neonatal nurses and midwives may feel that these approaches
shed little light on decision-making in difficult situations. Ethical

decision-making is now included in nursing and midwifery programmes of education, and study days are devoted to the topic, so basic ethical theory is accessible to all. It is then up to individual practitioners to examine the arguments for each standpoint and to reach a position with which they are comfortable and from which they can argue on behalf of the baby and the family.

THE EXTREMELY LOW BIRTH WEIGHT BABY

Case study

Jan C was admitted to the labour ward in advanced labour at 23 weeks gestation. This was her fourth pregnancy, the others having ended in miscarriages before 20 weeks. At 43 she felt time was running out for her to achieve a successful outcome and was desperate for this baby to survive. She was seen by the consultant obstetrician who told the couple that, if the baby was delivered immediately, its chances of survival were so poor that the regional neonatal unit would not consider collecting it. The hospital's own special care unit would not be able to offer more than basic care to the baby. Despite the couple's pleas for everything possible to be done, when the baby was born, weighing 500 g, he was wrapped in a blanket and given to his parents to cuddle until he died about half an hour later.

Treatment of low birth weight babies

The question of what treatment should be offered to very small or very immature babies is one of the ethical issues that confronts midwives and nurses working in delivery suites and neonatal intensive care units. Only in the last two decades has it been possible to contemplate the survival of babies born at such extremes of size or gestation. There are documented cases of very tiny babies surviving at home wrapped in cotton-wool and nursed beside the fire (Vaux 1986) but these were the exception rather than the rule. In the majority of cases nature took its course, the baby died and the parents did not expect otherwise. Now technology exists to keep alive those who would otherwise die and the media fascination with these 'miracle babies' means that the public expects that every live-born baby should be given all available help.

However, survival rates for babies weighing between 500 g and 750 g are only of the order of 35%, and for gestations between 24 and 26 weeks about 60%, while the incidence of severe impairment in survivors below 1000 g is about 15% in good intensive care units (Levene et al 2000). Ideally, this information should be sensitively discussed with the parents before delivery so that they can make an informed choice about the treatment they wish for their child. But, as the case study shows, this choice may be limited by local factors such as the availability of intensive care cots or the views of the paediatricians, and parents are not in a position to *insist* on treatment that a doctor is not prepared to offer.

Unfortunately, the decision over whether to resuscitate a small baby often falls to the junior doctor who is called to the delivery. It is helpful if clear guidelines exist about when resuscitation should be attempted. Levene et al (2000) suggest that this should apply to all babies over 600 g and/or 24 weeks gestation or more, and for selected infants between 500 g and 600 g depending on history, condition at birth and parental wishes. They believe that babies of less than 24 weeks with fused eyelids are unlikely to survive and should be given to their parents to cuddle and allowed to die peacefully in their arms. However, for the midwife faced with the unexpected arrival of a very small baby it is best if every effort is made to maintain the baby in good condition until a decision is made by a senior paediatrician not to continue with resuscitation (EAP-RCPCH 1997). A cold, acidotic premature baby is at great risk of intraventricular haemorrhage, a major contributor to future disability, but if kept warm and oxygenated from the start a decision can always be made later not to proceed (Avery 1987). Where there is doubt as to gestation, the midwife should institute fetal monitoring in labour so that the baby has the best chance of being delivered in optimum condition (Avery 1987), although the parents should be warned that, when the time comes, resuscitation may not be appropriate.

WITHDRAWING INTENSIVE CARE

Case study

Baby Catherine was born at 26 weeks gestation to an unsupported mother with six other girls ranging in age from 2 to 16 years. By the time Catherine was 5 days old it was evident from brain scans that she had significant areas of brain damage. She was being ventilated and had some abnormal movements. The doctors suggested that intensive care treatment was no longer of benefit to Catherine and should, therefore, be discontinued but Catherine's mother became very distressed at this suggestion, saying that she did not want her baby killed.

Reasons for withdrawal of intensive care

Neonatal intensive care includes treatments such as assisted ventilation, total parenteral nutrition and exchange transfusion. Babies undergoing intensive care are overwhelmingly of low birth weight, but may also be term neonates with birth asphyxia, genetic conditions, infections or other illnesses. Adult survivors of intensive care have testified to the unpleasantness of the experience (Dunn 1982) and there is no reason to suppose it is any different for a baby. It must therefore be realised that there might be occasions when intensive care is doing more harm than good for a particular baby. If the eventual outcome for the baby is likely to be poor, discontinuing treatment should be seen as an option. This was the situation with baby Catherine, where the staff caring for her believed that prolonging her life was not in her best interests because of the probable degree of brain damage she had suffered. Debate usually centres on what constitutes a poor outcome and the importance of future 'quality of life'. Bissenden (1986) claims that the issue of the baby's future quality of life cannot be avoided. 'To suggest that a person who can achieve a physical and mental age of no more than 2, will remain totally dependent, and will be unable to communicate can have a good quality of life is wrong' (Bissenden 1986 p 640). This attitude would meet with sympathy from most quarters and the problem lies in confidently and accurately assessing the infant's prognosis and conveying it to the parents so that they can participate in an informed decision.

For the preterm baby the greatest danger probably comes from intraventricular haemorrhage and periventricular leukomalacia, both of which are consequences of hypoxic episodes before or after birth. Intraventricular haemorrhage has an incidence of approximately 33% in babies of 1500 g or less (Levene et al 2000). Both these conditions can be diagnosed by ultrasound, and experience over a number of years has enabled a fairly accurate picture of long-term outcomes to be built based on the correlation of scan results with post-mortem findings and follow-up studies (Bissenden 1986). When a baby's scan picture is read in conjunction with assessment of its clinical condition, it becomes easier to make a prediction about the degree of impairment that the baby is likely to suffer and then for a decision to be made as to whether continued intensive care is appropriate.

The question then arises as to who should make the decision to withdraw intensive care. Some paediatricians and ethicists believe that the parents are the appropriate decision-makers (Weir 1984) and many parents share this belief. 'We believe that the responsibility is ours. We made the babies. Therefore the responsibility for them starts that day' (Scottish parents of a preterm baby interviewed by McHaffie 2001 p 107). An English parent of a premature baby who developed severe cerebral palsy shared this view:

> If a crisis in treatment does occur, we feel there should be more onus on an informed decision by parents about the next steps. However difficult and traumatic it is to decide to stop treatment, nothing can compare with the anguish that dominates the lives of parents with a severely handicapped child. (Doyle 1992 p 11)

However, many professionals would question whether the burden of decision-making should fall on the parents and worry that a parent may feel lifelong responsibility and guilt for deciding that treatment should be discontinued (Whyte 1989 p 35). Some parents share this view: 'We didn't want to make that decision because that would be a decision we'd have to live with for the rest of our lives—thinking that we'd just given up on her' (McHaffie 2001 p 107).

Evans and Levene (1998) believe that such decisions are medical ones and should be made by the consultant responsible for the baby's care. In North America, ethics advisory committees are sometimes involved in such decisions, providing a forum for the open discussion of issues and opinions and helping to educate nursing and medical staff about the moral aspects of their work (Nelson & Shapiro 1996), but Campbell et al (1988) are concerned that such committees may undermine what they see as the leadership role of the consultant in these situations.

Most people would concede that the parents have a part to play, although disagreeing about who should have the final say so, in practice, decisions are usually made by an informal 'committee' of those involved in caring for the baby. This includes both professionals and parents, acting in what they feel are the best interests of the baby, taking into account its present condition and the likely prognosis.

Should other factors be taken into account, such as the cost to the taxpayer of a severely handicapped child who requires special education and care and will make no contribution to society? Vaux (1986) calls this the 'ethics of necessity' and believes that economic considerations should never override the best interests of the child.

However, the cost of caring for a severely impaired child is not measured in monetary terms alone. The parents' relationship is often put under intolerable strain, older siblings may be relatively neglected as their parents' time is taken up with the impaired child and further pregnancies may be shelved through fear of history repeating itself or simply because there is no time or energy left to cope with a new baby.

What should be the role of the neonatal nurse or midwife working in the neonatal unit or, indeed, caring for the mother? The Nursing and Midwifery Council (NMC) Code of Professional Conduct states that nurses and midwives should be 'personally accountable for ensuring that [they] promote and protect the interests and dignity of patients and clients' (NMC 2002). For neonatal nurses this means taking seriously their role as the baby's advocate, speaking on the child's behalf when decisions are being made and promoting what they see as its best interests. It is not necessarily a comfortable role. These nurses may find themselves in conflict with the doctors if they feel they are causing unnecessary suffering by continuing with intensive care or if they believe their decision to withdraw it is too hasty. They may also disagree with parents who withhold permission for certain treatments or, conversely, as with baby Catherine's mother, insist that they want everything possible done to keep their baby alive.

One vital role the nurse can fulfil is to ensure that the lines of communication are kept open between all parties so that feelings can be aired in an atmosphere of trust. The nurses caring for Catherine encouraged her mother to talk to her priest and, with her permission, involved him in discussions about Catherine's future. With time to think things through and repeated explanations, Catherine's mother eventually decided that her daughter had suffered enough. The ventilator was switched off and the family had a couple of hours together before Catherine died peacefully in her mother's arms.

Midwives caring for a mother on the postnatal ward can listen to what she is saying and familiarise themselves with what is happening to the baby in the neonatal unit. They can help the mother clarify her views, assist her in putting these over to those caring for the baby and offer support through a heartbreaking time. When all the views have been aired, someone has to take the responsibility for making the final decision and this is usually the consultant. Midwives and nurses then have an obligation to translate this into practice (Whyte 1989), ensuring that the baby continues to receive the highest standard of care and to help the family cope with the consequences of the decision.

KILLING OR LETTING DIE

Case study

Baby John was born at term by caesarean section following a placental abruption. He was severely asphyxiated, required ventilation and did not make any spontaneous respiratory effort. At 2 hours of age he began having fits, which were only controlled with large amounts of sedation. After several days the sedation was allowed to wear off so that John's neurological state could be assessed: the convulsions had stopped but John appeared to be comatosed. His parents were told that his outlook was very poor and that in view of this intensive care was no longer appropriate and it would be better to switch off the ventilator and allow John to die peacefully. They agreed to this; John was baptised, taken off the ventilator and given to them to hold. Unexpectedly, John began to breathe on his own. After a couple of days it became apparent that he was not going to die, although he remained very floppy and unresponsive. When there was no improvement after several weeks it was decided to remove John's nasogastric tube and only offer feeds if he cried. As John's parents watched him become thinner and dehydrated they asked if he could be given something to put him and them out of their misery.

How to treat the dying baby

In many cases, once the baby is taken off the ventilator death will ensue in a matter of hours or even minutes. This gives the parents valuable time to cuddle the baby, take photographs of the whole family together and gain memories that can assist later in their grieving. For the nurse it is an opportunity to retrieve some of the futility of the situation by helping the family through a grieving process that, if handled skilfully, can leave them stronger and closer. One American nurse summed up her feelings thus:

> If there is no progress and in fact the kid is getting worse, isn't it better to let him die with some semblance of dignity and then spend your time with the family, helping them to cope and get on with life? I try to help them find a meaning and a purpose in their child's life no matter how short or miserable it may have been ... Maybe even looking into the future, things they can do to remember this baby and changes they can make in future pregnancies to prevent the same situation from recurring. (Raines 1993 p 46)

However, if the baby is not tiny and immature but is larger with an abnormality or birth asphyxia, switching off the ventilator may not result in death swiftly following. What principles should govern the caring for these babies when survival is not desired but is likely if normal nursing care is given? This is perhaps one of the hardest situations to deal with in neonatal intensive care and is a cause of considerable stress to all those involved.

While the withdrawal of mechanical life support may be seen as acceptable 'letting die', active measures to end the baby's life would constitute euthanasia, which is illegal in the UK. But this can seem like the worst of all possible outcomes, namely a slow and distressing death or the survival of a baby with severe impairments. In the end a decision may have to be taken about whether tube-feeding is continued or not for, as Callahan put it: 'denial of nutrition may in the long run become the only effective way to make certain that ... biologically tenacious patients actually die' (Rothenberg 1986 p 227). In a review of medical literature on the subject Rothenberg (1986) found that warmth, hygiene, food and fluids were normally considered to be part of basic care, while artificially supplied fluids or nutrition, via an intravenous infusion or nasogastric tube for example, were seen by some as treatment and in a similar category as ventilation (BMA 2002). In the case of a preterm baby or a term baby with brain damage where there is no sucking reflex, not to give feeds via a nasogastric tube may be equivalent to starving that child to death. Many nurses find this morally unacceptable (Lowes 1993) and it rarely leads to an easy and dignified death, as the case of baby John illustrates. Each nurse and midwife needs to study the issues involved and decide on their own position, as there are no hard and fast rules in these situations (Rothenberg 1986). Doctors may ask for feeds to be withheld and, legally, nurses can follow this instruction without compromising their professional position (Lowes 1993), but they have to look after the baby day by day and deal with the parents' anguish as they watch their child become dehydrated and wasted.

This is a situation that is best discussed openly with attempts made to formulate a care plan for the baby that truly meets all the child's needs and is acceptable to the majority of the carers. Whyte (1989) hopes that 'with a team approach to care, nurses will be free to contribute to decision-making without fear of victimisation if they appear to be swimming against the tide' (p 67).

The question of analgesia and sedation also causes concern in relation to the baby who is dying. Unlike an adult, babies cannot say when they are in pain or distress and it therefore becomes the responsibility of their carers to decide when treatment is required. Nurses who readily administer pain relief to babies postoperatively may be reluctant to do so if this may shorten the baby's life and there is little evidence of pain. Again, this situation needs to be aired openly and an acceptable course of action determined.

THE BABY WITH IMPAIRMENTS

Case study

Baby Shane was born at 34 weeks with Down's syndrome. He was the first baby of a couple in their 20s. He was also found to have oesophageal atresia and a severe cardiac defect. The paediatric surgeon advised that his postoperative prognosis would be poor, even if he survived surgery, and was reluctant to operate. The neonatologist agreed and Shane was given 'tender loving care' on the neonatal unit by his parents and the staff until he died at 10 days old.

How to treat the baby with impairments

With the increased use of antenatal screening tests and ultrasound in pregnancy, fewer babies with serious impairments are being delivered. Conditions that can be detected in early pregnancy and for which termination may be offered include spina bifida, hydrocephalus, polycystic kidneys, Down's syndrome and other chromosomal and genetic abnormalities. The birth of a baby with one of these abnormalities, undetected during the antenatal period, may come as even more of a shock to both parents and staff than one anticipated after a positive blood or scan result. In some cases the defect is incompatible with survival beyond a few days and the parents can be given a firm prognosis and helped to cope with their infant's short life expectancy.

However, in other cases, in fact with most of the conditions listed, the baby may survive for years with or without surgical or other active treatment. A decision has to be made as to whether, and how much, treatment will promote a good quality of life. The selection for surgery of only those babies whose quality of life is likely to be improved by it has been common practice for many years. In the early 1970s Lorber, a paediatric surgeon in Sheffield, published a number of papers describing the results of treating only certain babies born with myelomeningocele (Weir 1984 p 67). Around the same time similar suggestions, that some babies with impairments should not be treated actively, were being published in the United States. Conditions mentioned in the North American papers included anencephaly, microcephaly, intestinal obstructions, severe birth asphyxia, Down's syndrome and spina bifida.

Other paediatricians on both sides of the Atlantic, writing in the 1970s, disagreed with these views. Zachary, a colleague of Lorber's, considered that the majority of babies born with spina bifida should be given the treatment necessary to minimise their disabilities, including surgery: 'I believe that our patients, no matter how young or small they are, should receive the same consideration and expert help that would be considered normal in an adult' (Zachary 1976 p 76). It was pointed out by others that an untreated infant who survived, and no one was able to say that withholding treatment always led to the baby's death, might suffer more impairment than if vigorously treated from the start (Weir 1984).

Legal cases resulted in differing outcomes. In England in 1981 Dr Arthur was charged with murder after he prescribed sedation and the withholding of feeds for a baby with Down's syndrome whose parents had rejected him. Public opinion about the case was divided but Dr Arthur was acquitted by the jury. In America in 1982 the parents of a baby with Down's syndrome, tracheo-oesophageal fistula and oesophageal atresia refused consent for surgery on the advice of their obstetrician. He then ordered the baby to be fed, knowing that this was likely to cause the baby's death from aspiration. When the nurses refused to carry out this instruction, lawyers acting for the baby sought a court order to authorise intravenous feeding. This was rejected and the baby (known as 'Baby Doe') subsequently died (Whyte 1989). The case provoked extensive public and medical debate and eventually resulted in the passing of legislation in 1985 to protect infants with impairments, the so-called 'Baby Doe' regulations. The 'withholding of medically indicated treatment from a disabled infant with a life-threatening condition' was prohibited unless it would merely prolong the act of dying and would not contribute to the infant's survival (Moreno 1987). Although this law did not require that all babies with impairments should be treated, there was, perhaps as a result of this legislation, a tendency to overtreatment by American paediatricians. A British television programme shown in February 1995 filmed a 2-year-old anencephalic baby in the United States being kept alive—at the insistence of her mother, backed up by court rulings—with nasogastric feeds and resuscitation when she stopped breathing (ITV 1995). In the UK there is no legal imperative that forces doctors to continue treatment which they consider futile, and where cases have been tested in the courts the medical judgement has normally been upheld (McHaffie 1998).

A combination of factors will generally determine what treatment is offered to a baby with impairments: the views of the neonatologist, the severity of the condition, the availability of surgical treatment, the views of the paediatric surgeon, the gestation of the infant and the parents' attitudes and beliefs.

To help with decisions about withholding and withdrawing life support the Ethics Advisory Committee of the Royal College of Paediatrics and Child Health published a Framework for Practice (EAC-RCPCH 1997). This describes a number of situations in which the withholding or withdrawal of 'curative medical treatment' from neonates might be considered. These include non-resuscitation of the baby with a congenital abnormality incompatible with survival, such as anencephaly; non-resuscitation of a baby born at 23 weeks gestation or less where survival would be associated with such severe neurological impairment that many weeks of intensive care could not be justified; and the withdrawal of ventilation from a baby who is shown to have profound brain damage. The guidelines stress that such decisions should have the agreement of the baby's parents and that withdrawal of curative treatment should signal the initiation of palliative care, with a care plan being devised that addresses all the baby's physical and emotional needs and those of the family. To ignore these needs is to convey the message that the impairment negates the value of the infant's life.

ETHICAL ISSUES IN THE ALLOCATION OF RESOURCES

Neonatal intensive care, in common with other critical care, is expensive. In 1984 Newns estimated the cost of a neonatal intensive care survivor of less than 1000 g to be £10 000; for babies who did not survive the mean cost was £1000 (Newns et al, 1984). However it can be argued that because of the potential lifespan of survivors, neonatal intensive care is relatively cheap. Where neonatal intensive care produces a child who will take its place in society, few would disagree that this is money well spent. It is when survivors require considerable help from the state in terms of special schooling or benefits that doubts are raised about the cost-effectiveness of neonatal units. As the NHS is increasingly expected to operate as a business, it can be anticipated that cost considerations will play a larger part in decisions about care.

The area of resources encompasses both staff and equipment and these are often in limited supply. Stories abound of parents who claim that their baby was taken off a ventilator to make room for another. While this is, in reality, probably a rare occurrence, it is true that insufficient intensive care cots exist for all the neonates who require them, and some form of rationing does have to be used. This may simply be a refusal to consider for treatment any baby below a given weight or gestation. A 'first-come-first-served' policy is also usual, which may mean that a larger, more mature baby (with a better chance of intact survival) cannot be accommodated because smaller and less mature babies are occupying the available cots and ventilators. It would usually be considered unethical to take one of these babies off the ventilator to make room for a baby with a better prognosis. But that latter baby is then denied any chance at worst or at best has to undergo the hazards of a longer journey to a unit with a space. The tendency is to try to squeeze the baby in, which can place unacceptable pressures on already stretched staff and jeopardise the care of all the other babies in the unit.

As the number of preterm multiple births increases as a result of fertility treatments (see Chapter 10), neonatal units could be faced with the problem of a set of triplets taking over a number of ventilators, stretching resources to the limit and giving one family several babies while perhaps denying others even one. The arrival of a set of preterm multiples is to a neonatal unit what a major incident is to a casualty department, except that the preterm babies will take up beds for many weeks. The fact that these babies have been conceived with difficulty makes the desire to save them stronger but places an immense strain on available resources.

CONCLUSION

Neonatal intensive care is a branch of nursing/midwifery that offers enormous rewards for those who work within it. To see a very immature baby leave for home with its parents after weeks of highly skilled care and then return months later apparently developing normally, makes all the hard work, tiredness and heat seem worthwhile. There is also satisfaction in helping a family through bereavement and knowing that everything possible has been done to help ease their pain and assist them to grieve. What makes neonatal intensive care practitioners question their role is when they hear that a baby on whom they lavished care for weeks has developed a major impairment, or when they are asked to continue to ventilate a baby who has suffered severe brain damage but is being denied a peaceful death.

If those working in neonatal intensive care units, both nursing and medical staff, can foster an atmosphere of trust and open discussion, many of the ethical difficulties can be eased or avoided. Formal or informal support networks can provide opportunities to share the load, both for those who have to make difficult decisions and for those who have to carry them out. Individual practitioners need to develop their own philosophy based on understanding and consideration of the issues involved, so that they can provide the best service for the babies and families in their care.

References

Avery G 1987 Ethical dilemmas in the treatment of the extremely low birth weight infant. Clinics in Perinatology 14:361–365

Bissenden J 1986 Ethical aspects of neonatal care. Archives of Disease in Childhood 61:639–641

British Medical Association (BMA) 2002 Withdrawing and withholding life prolonging therapy. BMA Books, London

Campbell A, Lloyd D, Duffty P 1988 Treatment dilemmas in neonatal care: who should survive and who should decide. Annals of New York Academy of Sciences 530:92–103

Doyle C 1992 Dominic and the ethical tightrope. The Daily Telegraph, London, 1 September

Dunn A 1982 The human factor. Nursing Times 78:471

Ethics Advisory Committee/Royal College of Paediatrics and Child Health (EAC-RCPCH) 1997 Withholding or withdrawing life saving treatment in children. Royal College of Paediatrics and Child Health, London

Evans D, Levene M 1998 Ethical and legal dilemmas in the late management of severely damaged neonates without extensive brain damage. Seminars in Neonatology 3:285–290

ITV 1995 3D 16 February

Kuhse H, Singer P 1985 Handicapped babies: a right to life? Nursing Mirror 160:17–20

Lee R, Morgan D (eds) 1989 Birthrights: law and ethics at the beginnings of life. Routledge, London

Levene M, Tudehope D, Thearle, M J 2000 Essentials of neonatal medicine, 3rd edn. Blackwell Scientific Publications, Oxford

Lowes L 1993 Ethical decision-making: theory to practice. Paediatric Nursing 5:10–11

McHaffie H 1998 Withdrawing treatment from neonates: a review of the issues. British Journal of Midwifery 6(6): 384–388

McHaffie H 2001 Crucial decisions at the beginning of life. Radcliffe Medical Press, Oxford

Moreno J 1987 Ethical and legal issues in the care of the impaired newborn. Clinics in Perinatology 14:345–360

Nelson R, Shapiro R 1996 The role of an ethics committee in resolving conflict in the neonatal intensive care unit. Neonatal Intensive Care 9:26–30, 54

Newns B, Drummond M, Durbin G et al 1984 Costs and outcomes in a regional neonatal intensive care unit. Archives of Disease in Childhood 59:1064–1067

Nursing and Midwifery Council (NMC) 2002 Code of conduct. Online. Available: www.nmc-uk.org

Raines D 1993 Deciding what to do when the patient can't speak. Neonatal Network 12(6):43–48

Ramsey P 1982 Introduction. In: Horan D, Delahoyde M (eds) Infanticide and the handicapped newborn. Brigham Young University Press, Provo, UT

Rothenberg L S 1986 To feed or not to feed: that is the question and the ethical dilemma. Journal of Paediatric Nursing 1:226–229

Vaux K L 1986 Ethical issues in caring for tiny infants. Clinics in Perinatology 13(2):477–484

Walters J W 1988 Approaches to ethical decision making in the neonatal intensive care unit. American Journal of Diseases in Childhood 142:825–830

Weir R 1984 Selective non treatment of handicapped newborns. Oxford University Press, Oxford

Whyte D A 1989 Ethics in neonatal nursing. In: Brykcznska G M (ed) Ethics in paediatric nursing. Chapman and Hall, London

Wyatt J 1998 Matters of life and death. Inter-Varsity Press, London

Zachary R 1976 The neonatal surgeon. British Medical Journal 2:86–70

Chapter **8**

Screening and the perfect baby

Janet Holt

CHAPTER CONTENTS

INTRODUCTION

Screening and diagnostic tests to detect fetal abnormality are available to most women as part of prenatal care and major advances in the field of prenatal diagnosis have been achieved in the last 20 years. The use of diagnostic tests is becoming more common, it is possible to detect more diseases and the tests themselves have become more accurate as old techniques are refined and new ones developed. These advances have been made possible by improved medical technology but, as in so many other areas of health care where technology plays a vital role, ethical questions inevitably arise. The precise incidence of congenital abnormalities is difficult if not impossible to define. Many early spontaneous abortions are thought to be the result of abnormalities in the fetus, while other abnormalities may not be detected during pregnancy and may remain unrecognised until some time after birth. Congenital abnormalities are, however, relatively rare, with an estimated figure of about 3% of all fetuses having a major malformation (Eisenberg & Schenker 1997).

The aim of prenatal diagnosis is to detect congenital and genetic conditions in the fetus, which can be classified into two main groups. Some are genetic abnormalities responsible for conditions such as Huntingdon's disease, thalassaemia or cystic fibrosis and tests may be offered to women when there is a known family history. The other group of congenital abnormalities includes neural tube defects and Down's syndrome, which are not genetic defects, but certain women are known to be more at risk than others of having an affected fetus. Screening programmes have been developed at local and national levels to detect such conditions and abnormalities. If abnormalities are detected the diagnosis can be useful in three ways. First, the information allows parents to prepare both physically and psychologically for the birth of their baby. Second, it may be possible to instigate some form of treatment to correct the disease or abnormality either in utero or following delivery, and early diagnosis allows arrangements to be made. Finally, termination of the pregnancy may be considered. Although the practice of prenatal diagnosis encompasses all three purposes, Bewley (1994) alleges that 'termination currently dominates management' (p 1), while Abramsky (2000) considers the detection of an abnormality in the fetus as the first step towards the woman being offered the option of terminating the pregnancy.

Prenatal care allows screening for fetal abnormality using a variety of methods. An ultrasound scan is routinely offered to women around 18 weeks gestation. A scan at this stage of pregnancy is useful because, as well as detecting structural abnormalities, the fetus can be measured to confirm the expected date of delivery, multiple pregnancies can be identified and the location of the placenta determined. Advances in the use of transvaginal probes has allowed ultrasound screening to take place in the first 12 weeks of pregnancy, but this technique has not as yet replaced the 18-week scan. Serum screening used to identify blood biochemical markers of Down's syndrome is commonly offered to women at 16 weeks gestation, but the selection of women to be offered the test varies from hospital to hospital. Serum screening gives women an individual predicted risk of having a baby with Down's syndrome, but cannot indicate if the fetus is definitely affected by Down's syndrome or not. Any woman considered to be high risk can then be offered amniocentesis, where a sample of amniotic fluid is withdrawn, and fetal cells within it cultured and examined, allowing an accurate diagnosis to be made. Some centres offer chorionic villus sampling (CVS), a technique that allows specimens of placental tissue to be taken and examined to identify chromosomal abnormalities. Both amniocentesis and CVS are invasive procedures that carry an associated 1% risk of spontaneous abortion, but research is being carried out to develop non-invasive methods of assessing fetal well-being without compromising the fetus (Miller & Cuckle 2001). Preimplantation genetic diagnosis is a relatively new technique offered to couples who have previously had a child affected by a genetic defect, or who have terminated a pregnancy following diagnosis of an affected fetus. Embryos produced by in vitro fertilisation are tested for genetic defects, and only non-affected embryos are implanted into the uterus. The Human Fertilisation and Embryology Authority strictly regulates the use of preimplantation genetic diagnosis in the United Kingdom, and currently only five centres are licensed to perform it. As only healthy embryos are implanted, abortion is avoided.

It could be argued that prenatal diagnosis, with its emphasis on detecting fetuses with abnormalities, lies more in the province of obstetrics than midwifery and is therefore not of concern to midwives. While this may be true, midwives caring for women in pregnancy may find themselves involved in the prenatal diagnostic process in different ways. For example, a midwife may provide information to the woman about the tests offered, may be present while blood is taken or an amniocentesis performed, or may care for and deliver a woman undergoing a termination of pregnancy. It would therefore be difficult for midwives not to encounter some aspect of prenatal diagnosis in their practice, either directly or indirectly. It is obvious that midwives need to be knowledgeable about the tests available and the procedures for carrying out these tests, but they should also be aware of the ethical questions raised by the practice of prenatal diagnosis.

Many ethical questions arise as a result of using prenatal diagnosis, the most obvious one surrounding the decision to terminate the pregnancy when an impairment is detected, but there are other problems to consider; for example, how abnormality or impairment is to be defined, how severe it must be to justify a termination of pregnancy, and for what conditions screening should be offered. There are obvious diseases and abnormalities such as cystic fibrosis and neural tube defects that can be screened for, and less tangible conditions such as a genetic predisposition to developing cancer. Are we simply seeking the 'perfect baby' and rejecting less than perfect fetuses, including those considered to be the wrong sex? What is the ethical justification for using screening programmes? Should health professionals be obliged to offer the tests to all women, or just those considered at risk? This chapter will attempt to address some of these issues by examining the justification for screening programmes and the moral and legal status of the fetus. What constitutes an abnormality; the implications for existing people with impairments and the issues of eugenics and designer babies will be explored, with particular reference to the 'slippery slope' argument.

PRENATAL SCREENING PROGRAMMES

It is impractical to offer a comprehensive service to every pregnant woman to test for all potential abnormalities. Even if this were possible, there is a danger that the fetus would be exposed to a greater risk of miscarriage as a result of the tests, than the chances of an abnormality being detected. Use of prenatal diagnosis therefore tends to be restricted to individuals considered to be at high risk. For example, serum screening may be offered to women followed by amniocentesis if the test shows a high risk that the fetus is affected by Down's syndrome, but the test is not necessarily offered to all pregnant women. Wald et al (1998) describe the screening service in Britain as fragmented and incomplete, claiming that 'current screening practice in Britain is inequitable, with access to established screening tests being dependent on area of residence, and in some areas, a woman's age' (p 89). Individual hospital trusts and health authorities have differing criteria and while some may offer the test to all women, others restrict its use to those considered to be at high risk. While this may be justified on economic grounds by balancing the cost of screening programmes against risk, based, for example, on maternal age, it is not clear how such practices can be morally justified.

The use of screening programmes to detect abnormalities can be justified by taking a consequentialist approach to what constitutes a right or wrong action. In this view, the action itself is not inherently right or wrong, but what is important is the consequence of performing the action. The consequentialist will act to try to produce the best consequences for all concerned, which in this situation includes the pregnant woman, her partner, existing children and society in general. If the birth of healthy babies is preferred and the birth of babies with some form of disability is to be avoided, then to maximise preferences women at risk of having a baby with an impairment should be offered prenatal diagnostic tests. This may result in the abortion of an affected fetus, which, it may be argued, is a bad action, but such an action can be justified if more favourable consequences, such as the birth of healthy babies, are achieved. An example of a widely available screening programme is the one that aims to detect fetuses with Down's syndrome.

The risk of having a child with Down's syndrome rises considerably when the woman is over 35 years old and women in this age group are routinely offered tests to detect Down's syndrome. While it is more common today for women over the age of 35 to become pregnant, the total number of births in women over the age of 35 is less than in younger age groups. Precisely because of the introduction of prenatal screening programmes, most babies with Down's syndrome are born to women under the age of 35 who, because of differences in service provision, may not have been routinely offered prenatal diagnosis. So even if it were possible to screen 100% of pregnant women over 35 and ensure that all affected fetuses were aborted, a considerable number of fetuses with Down's syndrome would go undetected. This is because some women may not have been considered personally at risk and consequently may not have been offered any diagnostic tests. Although this provides a useful service for the individual, it is inconsistent with the broader consequentialist justification for screening programmes. If the birth of babies with Down's syndrome is to be avoided in society as a whole, then screening programmes need to be available to all women, not just those considered personally at risk.

THE MORAL AND LEGAL STATUS OF THE FETUS

One of the most fundamental ethical problems in prenatal diagnosis is the link with the option of induced abortion. Opinions vary widely about the morality of abortion in general, ranging from the extreme conservative position that disapproves of abortion in any circumstances, to the extreme liberal position that supports abortion in any circumstances. Between these two extremes are a multitude of other opinions on the morality of abortion, particularly concerning pregnancy due to rape, the period of gestation when the abortion is to be carried out, the risk of pregnancy to the mother's health and fetal abnormality. For example, some argue that abortion should not be generally available, but may be used in certain specific circumstances such as cases of fetal abnormality. This type of argument seems to suggest that abortion on these grounds differs from other types of abortion and is morally defensible.

The Abortion Act 1967 amended by section 37 of the Human Fertilisation and Embryology Act 1990 states that abortion is lawful if the pregnancy is less than 24 weeks advanced and the continuation of the pregnancy involves a risk of injury to the physical or mental health of the woman or of her existing children that is greater than if the pregnancy were terminated. However the Act considers abortion on the grounds of fetal abnormality separately and permits abortion at any stage in the pregnancy when there is 'substantial risk that if the child were born it will suffer from such physical or mental abnormalities as to be seriously handicapped'. What this means is that abortion in the vast majority of cases is only lawful when performed under 24 weeks gestation, but in instances where fetal abnormality is detected there is no such time limit. This suggests that in law at least, abortion performed on the grounds of fetal abnormality is viewed differently from other sorts of abortion.

Opinion may be similarly divided over the morality of abortion in general, and also there are opposing views about whether abortion for fetal abnormality is ethically different from abortions given for other reasons. These views can be considered from the position of the fetus, the parents and society in general. The opinion of the fetus may seem irrelevant as it cannot be said to be a self-conscious being, but as the fetus will develop into a child with some sort of impairment it may be suggested that if the child is likely to experience a life of suffering, disadvantage or discrimination then it would be better not to be born at all. In the United States some disabled people have initiated legal proceedings against their parents for not aborting them when fetal abnormality was detected in pregnancy. In the UK, the Court of Appeal in *McKay v Essex AHA* (1982) dismissed such a claim for wrongful life (Fletcher et al 1995).

Use of preimplantation diagnosis avoids the need for abortion, and may be attractive for those who consider the value of the fetus to increase throughout pregnancy. According to this view, the failure to select an embryo for implantation is morally preferable to aborting a more developed fetus later in pregnancy. The practice will however be as unacceptable as abortion at any stage of pregnancy for those who believe that life begins at conception. In this view, the moral status of the embryo is not understood to be different to that of the more developed fetus, new born baby or even an adult.

Preimplantation diagnosis can, however, raise other ethical difficulties. It is most commonly used to detect single gene defects such as cystic fibrosis and chromosome abnormalities. In some sex-linked disorders such as Duchenne muscular dystrophy, however, the identification of the genetic condition at this molecular level is not possible, but the sex of the embryo can be determined and only embryos of the sex unaffected by the disorder selected for implantation. It may be argued that while the detection of affected or potentially affected embryos is of benefit to the woman, her partner and existing children, concerns have been expressed about the use of sex-selection purely on the basis of a preference for one sex or the other. Likewise, some people object to the idea of 'saviour siblings', where an embryo with a certain tissue type is implanted to enable the treatment of an existing child (see later). Those who think that embryos are less morally signifi-cant than fetuses, as well those who think that moral significance begins with conception, may object to selection for these reasons.

Justifications for abortion in the case of fetal abnormality often require difficult calculations to be made about how much suffering might render a life not worth living, which abnormalities might be associated with such a poor quality of life, and the extent to which different abnormalities are likely to disadvantage the child or adult in later life. It is easy to distinguish between the anencephalic fetus (who will die shortly after birth because there is no possible treatment) and the fetus with a cleft lip (a condition that can be successfully treated with surgery following delivery). Whereas an anencephalic fetus has little to gain from being born (lacking any capacity for consciousness, including any capacity to experience pleasure or even pain), the fetus with the cleft lip is not facing a lifetime of suffering or disadvantage. Far more complex are conditions such as Down's syndrome that affect individuals in many different ways. Some children with Down's syndrome have multiple abnormalities or profound learning difficul-ties and are unable to perform even the simplest tasks. Others receive mainstream education, become employed and form all the usual social relationships. Using prenatal diagnosis, it is not possible to detect or predict what sort of effects Down's syndrome will have on the child or adult in later life nor, therefore, to argue with confidence that a termination will prevent a lifetime of suffering.

In the majority of cases the results of prenatal diagnostic tests are not available in the early stages of pregnancy. For many women, the pregnancy has been planned or accepted and abortion is not an option under consideration. Following prenatal diagnosis, women (and their partners) may be faced with the decision whether to continue with or to terminate the pregnancy. Research seems to suggest that when the prognosis is poor, most women decide on termination of the pregnancy. For example, a systematic literature review carried out by Mansfield et al (1999) showed the termination rate to be 92% after prenatal diagnosis of Down's syndrome, and 64% following a diagnosis of spina bifida. The birth of a child with a disability may have profound effects on a family, and the decision to continue with the pregnancy or not will have to be made taking such factors into consideration. The parents' view about the right thing to do may depend on their attitudes to abortion in general, their conception of abnormality and their understanding of disability. In a paper examining the concept of abnormality, Hoedemaekers & Ten Have (1999) describe the term abnormality as 'frequently used, but seldom explained' (p 537). They query the standards used to judge a specific condition, function or structure as abnormal or normal, and argue that the precise role of value judgements in the decision-making process is obscure. For some individuals making a judgement about what constitutes an abnormality may be difficult or impossible because they have no experience of the condition in question, but it can be no less difficult for those who do have this experience. In a study of 78 parents of Down's syndrome children, there was disagreement among the parents about what constituted a severe impairment. For one woman in this study, having had a child classed as 'handicapped' had altered her idea of what being handicapped really was (Shepherdson 1983).

Ultimately parents may make a decision to terminate a pregnancy based on a reluctance to give birth to a child who will potentially face a life of suffering or discrimination. But is this really the case? Do children or adults with an impairment and their carers experience miserable lives? If fetuses with impairments are aborted, is there an underlying assumption that they are less valuable than 'normal' fetuses and if so what are the implications of this for existing people with impairments?

IMPLICATIONS FOR EXISTING PEOPLE WITH IMPAIRMENTS

Not all children and adults with an impairment have a genetic condition, but a proportion are affected because of genetic disease or abnormal embryonic or fetal development. Some will be affected because of an abnormality that could have been detected in pregnancy and selective abortion carried out. There may be many reasons why people have been born with impairments rather than aborted as fetuses. It may be that screening tests were not available to their mothers, or that their mothers were not considered to be at high risk, or that abortion was rejected as an option. If selective abortion for fetal abnormality can be justified, then we may want to ask if this will alter the attitude of society towards those with impairments. Could it be that people with impairments whose birth could have been prevented by the use of prenatal diagnosis and selective abortion may be considered less valuable and not given access to social and medical facilities?

Provisions to prevent people with impairments becoming disabled are positively encouraged: new buildings are designed for use by those using wheel chairs, old buildings are adapted as necessary, and theatres and television use sign language and subtitles for those with hearing impairments; many job advertisements carry a statement encouraging applications from disabled people; and in the UK the Disability Discrimination Act 1995 protects the rights of disabled people. Instead of shutting people with learning difficulties away from the rest of society in institutions, there has been a shift towards care in the community. It seems obvious that people with special needs should have these needs met with a view to minimising restrictions on their lifestyle caused by these needs. This seems to be inconsistent, however, with the way that impairments are viewed when selective abortion is considered. If an abortion is carried out to prevent the birth of a child who faces life disadvantaged, this implies that it is better for that child not to be born rather than to be born with an impairment. But the reason that provisions are made for people with special needs is to improve the life of people with an impairment, and if this can be done it does not make sense to suggest that such a life is not worth living at all. Arguably, an increase in the use of selective abortion will marginalise those with an impairment still further so that even fewer provisions are made to meet their needs, which in its turn will compound the view that impairment inevitably leads to disability. Conversely, if there are fewer people with a disability in society then more could be done for them, as there would be fewer people competing for the same resources. While it is not clear how restricting prenatal diagnosis or abortion would improve the lives of existing people with impairments, Jackson (2000) argues that even if it did, forcing a woman to continue with a pregnancy against her wishes to achieve a shift in social attitudes would represent a marked exception (in law at least), to the current trend of regarding individual autonomy as the overriding consideration.

Irrespective of what tests and abortion facilities are offered to women in the future, it is unlikely that all genetic conditions will be eradicated either because, for some reason, the diagnosis was not made in pregnancy, or because some women refuse the option of selective abortion. It seems inconceivable that women, particularly in a democratic society, could be forced by law to have prenatal diagnostic tests and selective abortion if an impairment is found.

This issue was recognised by the Court of Appeal in *McKay v Essex AHA* (1982), which argued that imposing a duty to abort would infringe principles of sanctity of life and devalue disabled members of society in general (Fletcher et al 1995).

At present selective abortion is tolerated at the same time as measures are encouraged to improve the status of people with an impairment. One reason for this may be that there has not been a sharp decline in the number of babies born with genetic conditions, but rather this has been a more gradual process creating less of an impact on society. Regardless of this, researchers in the field of prenatal diagnosis aim to devise less invasive, less expensive tests that can be made available to more women, which in turn will doubtlessly further reduce the number of babies born with impairments. However, there is a distinction to be made between discrimination against the disabled and the negative effects of disability. Gillam (1999) argues that discrimination against people with impairments is not an objective or inevitable consequence of prenatal diagnosis, but this does not mean that potentially significant negative effects for existing people with an impairment do not exist. For example, quality of life assessments of a fetus found to have an impairment are likely to be closely connected with those made of people living with impairments, and judgements in the context of prenatal care probably made by someone with an outsider's view of disability. Although discrimination against people with an impairment, or the women who choose to carry to term rather than have a termination for fetal abnormality, is not officially sanctioned, we cannot be certain that this will be the case in the future. Economic constraints and increased financial demands on an already overburdened health care system will inevitably lead to questions being asked about the appropriate use of resources, particularly for those needing long-term care.

EUGENICS

Objections have been raised to prenatal diagnosis and selective abortion because its alleged 'seek and destroy' mission is a poorly disguised form of eugenics (Green et al 1992). In the late 19th century Francis Galton introduced the term eugenics from the Greek root meaning good in birth or noble in heredity. Galton intended to identify a science that improved human stock by giving 'the more suitable races or strains of blood a better chance of prevailing speedily over the less suitable' (Galton cited in Kelves 1985 p ix). However noble Galton's original intentions, eugenics is a controversial subject. It became associated with racist philosophies and the identification of individuals likely to indulge in criminal behaviour based on intelligence levels. The UK and the USA established eugenics societies and the sterilisation of people considered to be defective was permitted in some European countries and American states. The abuse of eugenics reached its peak during the Holocaust when millions of people with genetic profiles considered undesirable were murdered and eugenics as a science became discredited.

There are two types of eugenic theories, positive and negative. Negative eugenics attempts to identify inferior genes in a population and eliminate them to reduce the incidence of inferior characteristics. It may be argued that prenatal diagnosis is a form of negative eugenics as defective genes are identified and attempts are made to reduce the incidence of genetically inherited diseases and abnormalities. If these practices are a form of eugenics, then it may be plausible that they should be as morally suspect as previous practices. This suspicion is, however, dependent on an assumption that eugenic theories always have sinister applications, which is not necessarily the case. For example, soon after birth all babies are tested for phenylketonuria (PKU), an inherited disease that, if left untreated, causes severe learning difficulties. The test is relatively non-invasive, simple and inexpensive, but more importantly, the disease can be successfully treated by dietary restriction. This form of screening programme can be considered to be negative eugenics, as by identifying a disease caused by a defective gene, inferior characteristics, in this case learning difficulties, can be avoided. Clearly even the strictest opponents of eugenic theories would not object to this practice. The crucial issue here is that this practice benefits the child enormously because, although a defective gene is present, relatively simple treatment can be instigated to prevent profound impairments. Similarly, some people are aware of the fact that they have a family history of genetic diseases such as Huntingdon's disease, Tay–Sachs or cystic fibrosis. Prior to becoming pregnant the couple may attend genetic counselling sessions where the risks of the fetus being affected can be assessed. If there is a high risk, some couples may decide not to have a child. This practice can also be described as negative eugenics in that the birth of a child with such a condition is avoided, but again it is beneficial to the individuals if they choose not to have such a child. In both examples, defective genes are identified or attempts made to reduce the incidence of genetically inherited diseases and abnormalities, but in neither case is anyone killed.

Eugenics is a highly emotive subject because of its historical association with a quest to purify the gene pool, social cleansing and racist programmes and practices. While screening programmes to detect diseases like PKU are beneficial for individuals carrying the gene to avoid the impairments associated with the disease, the gene pool will not be improved unless individuals carrying the gene are prevented from having children. The gene pool could be improved more effectively if affected children were not only treated, but then sterilised to prevent them reproducing in the future. It would be even more effective to screen for as many inherited diseases as possible, even if treatments are not available, and sterilise the people affected to ensure that they too would be unable to have children with the same defective genes. Clearly the aim in testing babies for PKU or providing genetic counselling for couples with a family history of genetic disease is not an attempt to purify the gene pool but to offer services of great benefit to individuals, and as such they are not morally questionable. When such practices do become morally questionable is when they are abused, legally enforced or lead to other less desirable practices such as enforced sterilisation.

Selective abortion is described as an abuse of eugenics because abortion on such grounds is seen as analogous to the genocide practised by the Nazis. Although eugenics was central to the entire Nazi scheme, and it may be argued there are similarities between the two, it is not obvious that this is an appropriate analogy. The practice of genocide perpetrated by the Nazis was directed at improving the gene pool of the Aryan race on a national scale and people were forced to comply with the regulations. For women living in democratic societies, undergoing prenatal diagnosis and selective abortion is a decision that individuals make for personal reasons without force and not to comply with any regulations. Although a form of negative eugenics, it is possible to apply eugenic theories in ways that benefit society without any sinister undertones. Nevertheless, there still remains the possibility that these practices may be abused by forcing people to abort an abnormal fetus, by society adopting negative attitudes to people with impairments, or by trying to create the perfect designer baby.

DESIGNER BABIES

The questions raised by the creation of so-called designer babies are illustrated by two cases that received extensive media coverage in 2000. In the United States, following the birth of a child with Fanconi anaemia, Lisa and Jack Nash used preimplantation diagnosis to select an embryo that was not only free of the disease, but also one that had the correct tissue match for his affected sister. Following delivery, in a procedure unlikely to cause him any physical harm, stem cells collected from his umbilical cord were given to his sister to replace her bone marrow (Josefson 2000). The central question in this case concerned the motivation behind Mr and Mrs Nash's decision. Clearly they did not wish to have another child with a life-threatening condition, an understandable decision given their daughter's experience, but doubts were raised over their real desire to have another child other than as a donor to treat their daughter. Was the baby created for his own sake or only as a means to treat his sister? The creating of one child to provide tissue for another is morally questionable if this was the sole reason for having the child. If, for example, following removal of the stem cells, Mr and Mrs Nash had offered the baby for adoption, it would be fair to assume that their only interest in having the child was as a donor for their daughter. However, as the parents of one affected child, Mr and Mrs Nash could legitimately request preimplantation diagnosis to ensure they did not have an affected child, irrespective of the tissue match. It is plausible that their decision may have been motivated by a desire to produce two benefits from the procedure by having both an unaffected child and one with a suitable tissue type. This would suggest, therefore, that the baby was wanted and was not considered by his parents less valuable than his sister. Indeed it may be argued that precisely because of the benefits the baby has brought to his sister, his parents may consider him to be an exceptionally valuable and wanted child. The importance of identifying the parents' motives in using preimplantation diagnosis was demonstrated in two cases considered by the Human Fertilisation and Embryology Authority (HFEA) in 2002.

In the first case, the parents of Zain Hashmi, a child with the inherited condition beta thalassaemia, applied to use preimplantation diagnosis to select not only an unaffected embryo, but also one likely to be a suitable tissue match to treat their son. The HFEA granted permission for this to take place. In the second case, the parents of a Charlie Whittaker, a child with the rare condition Diamond Blackfan anaemia applied to use preimplantation diagnosis. In this case the child had not inherited the condition from his parents, and the HFEA rejected the application on the grounds that preimplantation diagnosis was not being used to prevent another child with this condition from being born, but being used solely to provide a compatible donor for their child. This, they argued, did not meet the HFEA's criterion that the embryos should themselves be at risk of the condition affecting the existing child. While the HFEA distinguished between the two cases and judged that the Hashmis' case fell within their criteria but the Whittaker's case did not, English et al (2002) question whether this is sufficient to constitute a moral distinction. In other situations embryos are created solely for research purposes, for example to improve fertility treatment and contraception. The use of an embryo to treat a child with a life-threatening disease seems to be at least equally appropriate. Debate of the moral questions brought into focus by these two cases is likely to continue and to be subject to further legal challenges.

The motives of Alan and Louise Masterton, a couple with four sons, who wanted to use preimplantation diagnosis to select a female embryo following the death of their only daughter, were also considered relevant to determining the permissibility of their request. The Human Fertilisation and Embryology Act 1990 prohibits sex selection for other than medical reasons, and the Mastertons' application was rejected by the HFEA (Josefson 2000). Clearly Mr and Mrs Masterton were motivated by a desire to have another child, but unlike the Nash and Hashmi cases, this cannot be explained in terms of a dual motivation. The baby would not be providing potentially life-saving treatment for a sibling, but was, according to the Mastertons, wanted as an addition to their family. However, doubts were expressed about whether Mr and Mrs Masterton wanted the baby for its own sake or only as a substitute for the daughter they had lost. While it seems exceptionally difficult to determine exactly what their motives were, even if they did view the child as a substitute, this does not necessarily mean that their second daughter would have been any less valuable to them than their first. As in the Nash and Hashmi cases, it may be argued that the baby would have been considered more valuable because of the difficulties encountered in her conception. However, even if it could somehow be shown beyond any doubt that this child was a wanted and valuable individual, the difficulties of selecting an embryo on the grounds of gender raises complex ethical questions.

The Ethics Committee of the American Society of Reproductive Medicine (1999) suggests there are several undesirable consequences of sex selection, such as inappropriate control of non-essential characteristics of children, risks of psychological harm to sex-selected children, potential changes in the human sex ratio, and inappropriate use of limited medical resources. Likewise, there is a danger that gender bias in society as a whole may be reinforced, particularly in societies that give preference to males. But as Wertz & Fletcher (1998) suggest, there is also the possibility of harm in cultures that prefer gender balanced families because it may perpetuate gender stereo-typing. However, modern prenatal diagnostic techniques, particu-larly preimplantation diagnosis, have made sex selection a reality, and while such techniques remain strictly regulated in the UK and elsewhere, requests such as those made by the Nashs, Mastertons, Hashmis and Whittakers are likely to occur and existing legislation will be challenged. The HFEA has recently carried out a public con-sultation exercise on sex selection, which is due to report in 2003. Sex selection is currently only permitted to avoid serious sex-linked genetic conditions, but the consultation document asks if this prac-tice should be available for non-medical reasons such as those raised in the Masterton case (HFEA 2002). It may be argued that although prenatal diagnosis and preimplantation diagnosis is not in itself morally questionable, by allowing the practice we may progress down a slippery slope that will culminate in morally dubious prac-tices in the future.

THE SLIPPERY SLOPE

This argument is frequently used by opponents of prenatal diagnosis and alleges that if one practice is allowed, then there will be a natural progression to other practices. Williams (1985) has described two different forms of the slippery slope argument: the 'horrible result argument' and the 'arbitrary result argument'. The 'horrible result' argument concentrates on what is at the bottom of the slope. Although the practice of prenatal diagnosis itself can be morally justified, there is a danger of a natural progression towards practices that are not. For example, detection of an anencephalic fetus may be morally permis-sible, but allowing selective abortion of the anencephalic fetus may subsequently lead to the detection and abortion of a fetus for less acceptable reasons such as being the wrong gender, or having the wrong physical characteristics or IQ. Supporters of this argument would suggest that the only way to ensure that society does not slide down the slippery slope towards this horrible result is not to allow prenatal diagnosis or selective abortion in the first place.

This argument may be significant because there have been clear cases of abuse in the past. We know that it is possible for abusive practices to occur and the memories of these past events are all too apparent. However, it may be argued that precisely because such abuses are remembered, then this memory in itself may serve to make people aware of the potential dangers and thereby prevent the repetition of such practices. It is of course impossible to disinvent practices. Although it may be decided that there is a strong case for the prevention of prenatal diagnosis because of what this practice may lead to, the knowledge of prenatal diagnostic techniques will remain, along with the potential for misuse. Even if it were possible to do so, banning prenatal diagnosis and selective abortion could be counterproductive, as failing to regulate practices for which the techniques are known may lead to their covert use and misuse.

The 'arbitrary result argument' suggests that once on the slippery slope any further discrimination will be arbitrary. If it is deemed morally unacceptable to detect and abort a fetus because it is abnormal, then there is no slope leading to more arbitrary chosen characteristics being included. Alternatively, if this practice is considered to be morally acceptable, it becomes necessary to decide what constitutes an abnormality. As stated previously, fetal abnormalities range from being incompatible with life to what might be described as minor physical defects, with a wide range of variations in between. If an abnormality incompatible with life is detected, then there may seem little point in continuing with the pregnancy and so a distinction could be made between these cases and others. There are other situations when the outcome cannot be so clearly defined, as for example in cases of spina bifida. Sometimes the abnormality is severe and the baby will die soon after birth, but in other cases the child may only be slightly affected or corrective surgery may be possible.

If prenatal diagnosis and selective abortion are allowed for some cases of fetal abnormality, then to draw the line between these and other abnormalities may seem to be arbitrary. In many areas of life we do resort to making arbitrary distinctions, such as the selection of 30 miles per hour as the speed limit for vehicles in residential areas. It may not be clear why this precise speed should be selected, but it is obvious that we should distinguish between safe and dangerous speeds for vehicles. Suppose that a policeman observes one person driving at 31 miles per hour and another driving at 29 miles per hour; he may fine the first person but not the second, a harsh action when the distinction is so small, but abolishing the speed regulations altogether is not a viable solution. In the same way it may be possible to distinguish between those abnormalities where detection and abortion would be permissible and those where it is not, for example between severe abnormalities and minor abnormalities but difficult borderline cases, like spina bifida, will remain. The existence of these difficult cases does not, however, mean that screening should be abandoned altogether.

CONCLUSION

There can be little doubt that the practice of prenatal diagnosis raises a multitude of ethical questions, particularly pertaining to selective abortion of abnormal fetuses. Abortion on grounds of fetal abnormality is not only legal, but the law governing abortion for abnormality is arguably more liberal than that permitting abortion in other circumstances. This does not, however, make the practice morally acceptable to everyone. Prenatal screening programmes can be justified using a consequentialist approach to ethics, but there is a tension between this justification and inequalities in the availability of tests. For some people screening programmes represent a quest for the perfect baby, are morally questionable, an application of negative eugenics theories and a practice that may have implications for the way that people with impairments are viewed in society. Undoubtedly tension exists between the current trend towards a more inclusive attitude towards people with impairments and aborting fetuses with the same conditions. At present, we appear to be able to tolerate such tensions, but against a backdrop of increasing demands on social and health care systems, we should not be confident that such positive attitudes will continue.

There are also concerns that, while in its current form prenatal diagnosis can be justified, we are poised at the top of a slippery slope towards less desirable practices: today it seems acceptable to abort a fetus with Down's syndrome and tomorrow it might seem just as acceptable to abort a fetus as a means of sex selection. While it has been argued that the most effective guard against a slippery slope is knowing that it is there, recent cases challenging existing legislation suggest that individuals are already pushing at the boundaries of what is currently acceptable. However, there is also a potential danger in not legislating to permit some use of prenatal screening; that is, it will drive the practice underground where it will be completely unregulated. This is a consequence unlikely to be of benefit either to women or to wider society.

References

Abramsky L 2000 Counselling patients undergoing prenatal tests and following the diagnosis of fetal abnormality. In: Twining P, McHugo J M, Pilling D W (eds) Textbook of fetal abnormalities. Churchill Livingstone, Edinburgh

Bewley S 1994 Ethical issues in prenatal diagnosis. In: Abramsky L, Chapple J (eds) Prenatal diagnosis. Chapman & Hall, London

Eisenberg V H, Schenker J L 1997 The moral aspects of prenatal diagnosis. European Journal of Obstetrics & Gynaecology 72:35–45

English V, Romano-Critchley G, Sheather J et al 2002 Born to be a donor? Journal of Medical Ethics, 28:384–385

Ethics Committee of the American Society of Reproductive Medicine 1999 Sex selection and preimplantation genetic diagnosis. Fertility and Sterility 72:595–598

Fletcher N et al 1995 Ethics, law and nursing. Manchester University Press, Manchester

Gillam L 1999 Prenatal diagnosis and discrimination against the disabled. Journal of Medical Ethics 25:163–171

Green J, Statham H, Snowdon C 1992 Screening for abnormalities: attitudes and experiences. In: Chard T, Richards T P M (eds) Obstetrics in the 1990s: current controversies. MacKeith Press, London, p 65–89

Hoedemaekers R, Ten Have H 1999 The concept of abnormality in medical genetics. Theoretical Medicine and Bioethics 20:537–561

Human Fertilisation and Embryology Act 1990 HMSO, London

Human Fertilisation and Embryology Authority 2002 Sex selection: choice and responsibility in human reproduction. HFEA, London

Jackson E 2000 Abortion, autonomy and prenatal diagnosis. Social and Legal Studies 9:467–494

Josefson D 2000 Couple select healthy embryo to provide stem cells for sister. British Medical Journal 321:917–918

Kelves D J 1985 The name of eugenics. Penguin Books, Harmondsworth

Mansfield C, Hopfer S, Marteau T M 1999 Termination rates after prenatal diagnosis of Down syndrome, spina bifida, anencephaly and Turner and Klinefelter syndromes: a systematic literature review. Prenatal Diagnosis 19:808–812

Miller D, Cuckle H S 2001 A needle in a haystack: prenatal diagnosis of Down's syndrome. Trends in Molecular Medicine 7:50

Shepherdson B 1983 Abortion and euthanasia of Down's syndrome children; the parent's view. Journal of Medical Ethics 9:152–157

Wald N J et al 1998 Antenatal screening for Down's syndrome. Health Technology Assessment 2(1)

Wertz D C, Fletcher J C 1998 Ethical and social issues in prenatal sex selection: a survey of geneticists in 37 nations. Social Science & Medicine 46:255–273

Williams B 1985 Which slopes are slippery? In: Lockwood M (ed) Moral dilemmas in modern medicine. Oxford University Press, Oxford, p 126–137

Chapter 9

Ethics of fetal tissue transplantation and research on embryos

David Lamb

INTRODUCTION

Debates over the legal and ethical regulation of transplants in the past 20 years have focused primarily on the adult and infant brain-dead donor. The use of tissues from aborted fetuses, and research on embryos and promordial germ cells raise a number of new legal and ethical issues. Does the fetus or embryo require special protection? Is a discarded fetus or embryo equivalent to other forms of 'medical waste'? What is the moral status of a fetus or embryo and whose consent should be sought for their use in research or therapy? Do existing statutes or codes of practice adequately regulate their retrieval? There are questions concerning the link between induced abortions and the use of fetal tissue derived from them. Can the potential benefits of fetal tissue transplantation be insulated from the moral taint of abortion, and to what extent do moral standpoints regarding abortion influence recent controversies over research on embryos? To what extent can the dead, aborted, fetus be regarded as morally equivalent to the brain-dead organ donor? Do the same arguments apply to discarded human embryos after IVF therapy? Or is the fetus or embryo to be regarded as a donatable organ or tissue comparable to a kidney or bone marrow? They cannot be both donors and donations. If, as some argue, they are morally equivalent to human beings, then they could be said to be donors, albeit 'involuntary' ones, but if they are donations, then their moral status is the same as that of organs and tissues.

These issues are of relevance to midwives as they may be involved in caring for a woman undergoing a pregnancy termination or a course of IVF therapy and may be required to help explain the choices the woman might have to make. Further debates concerning the moral status of the embryo or fetus are of central importance to midwives, as the attitude one adopts towards the embryo or fetus affects practice at every level.

The first part of this chapter will examine the ethical issues bound up with fetal tissue transplantation and the second part will examine some of the ethical issues bound up with research on human embryos and stem cells.

THE USE OF FETUSES AND FETAL TISSUE

Guidelines for the use of fetal material

The majority of commissions and investigative panels have concluded that the use of fetal tissue is ethical, provided that certain standards are in place. There have been over 20 reports from commissions and investigative panels worldwide on the use of fetal tissue and experimentation. Although different in minor respects (for example, there are different recommendations concerning the father's consent to the use of fetal tissue and different procedures for obtaining consent for the use of material after elected and spontaneous abortions), most of them have recommended that fetal tissue should be honoured with the respect accorded to dead bodies (Coutts 1993).

In the UK the Polkinghorne Committee, which reported in July 1989, outlined a Code of Practice that followed Sweden and the Netherlands in stressing the need for maternal consent. The committee also advocated a 'separation principle'; namely, that there must be 'a separation of the supply of fetal tissue from its use' (Polkinghorne 1989). Thus there must be no direct contact between abortion clinics and fetal tissue researchers. This was designed to ensure that the need for fetal tissue did not influence the decision to have an abortion. The Polkinghorne Committee (1989) took the view that:

> whatever one's ethical opinion about abortion itself, it does not
> follow that morally there is an absolute prohibition on the ethical use

of fetuses or fetal tissue from lawful abortion … the termination of pregnancy and the subsequent use of fetal tissue should be recognised as separate moral questions and we regard it as of great importance that the separation of these moral issues should be reflected in the procedures employed … great care should be taken to separate the decisions relating to abortion and the subsequent use of fetal material. The prior decision to carry out an abortion should be reached without consideration of the benefits of subsequent use.

According to the separation principle, informed maternal consent for tissue must be sharply separated from the decision to terminate the pregnancy. The Committee also recommended that the father's consent should not be required for the use of fetal material. The Polkinghorne Code of Practice was accepted by the Minister for Health and circulated to health authorities. It recommends that proposals to use fetal tissue for research and therapy must satisfy an ethics committee of the value of the research, indicate the absence of alternatives to the proposed use, and provide a demonstration that the researchers have the necessary facilities and skills to undertake the project.

Potential benefits of fetal tissue transplantation

In 1972 the Peel Report listed 53 ways in which research on fetal material could be of benefit (DHSS 1972). Since then there have been many more proposals that could be added to the list. The most immediate practical application of fetal tissue research is the transplantation of human fetal dopamine-secreting neurones to the brains of patients with Alzheimer's disease and medically unresponsive Parkinson's disease. The advantages of fetal material over other human tissue for transplantation purposes lie in its capacity to proliferate and its weak antigenicity. New applications are constantly sought. Recent use involves umbilical cells from fetuses as an alternative to bone-marrow transplantation, and research on fetal tissue could lead to therapies for infertility treatment and the prevention of many miscarriages.

Use of fetal tissue procured from legal and voluntarily undertaken abortions is justified with reference to the public good. Those who advocate the use of fetal tissue stress that abortions would not be performed in order to meet a need for human tissue; that the abortions would take place whether or not fetal remains were useful; that the material is better put to use for public benefit than destroyed;

and that material from whole or living fetuses is not requested, only aggregates of cells from dead fetuses (BMA 1988).

Despite the potential benefits of fetal tissue transplantation, a considerable number of ethical objections have been made, several of which will be examined here. It is also significant that many similar ethical objections have emerged in the controversy surrounding proposals for embryonic stem cell research, which will be examined in the second part of this chapter. The basic moral issue is not that new: it is partly bound up with the question as to whether certain human individuals can be exploited to provide benefits for others, and partly with deeply held beliefs regarding the level of respect due to bodily parts. There is an increasing awareness that the dead fetus should be treated with respect and piety, and that it is not equivalent to 'medical waste'. In the UK religious services are performed for dead fetuses and the Health Council of the Netherlands noted that it is common for the parents' desire for the cremation of a fetus to be recognised and respected (Health Council of the Netherlands 1994). The need to respect fetal remains is uncontested, as is evident in guidelines developed for dealing with the products of late abortion. Philosophers who disregard the moral status of the fetus, with abstruse appeals to criteria for personal identity, have not even begun to recognise the moral issues involved. The most powerful objection to the use of fetal tissue is bound up with the ongoing controversy over the rights and wrongs of voluntary abortion. The source of the controversy lies in the fact that the tissue involved is derived from induced abortion, the morality of which continues to generate religious and moral disagreement.

Abortion and the separation principle

Can discussions about the potential benefits of fetal tissue research and transplantation be morally insulated from arguments about the rights and wrongs of induced abortions? Or is it necessary to have reached the conclusion that voluntary abortion is ethically acceptable before one can advance arguments in favour of fetal tissue transplantation? These questions have so far dominated the debate on both sides of the Atlantic.

Objections to fetal transplants include the arguments that it promotes a degrading attitude to human beings, that killing and dissecting a fetus is a violation of the rights of the developing human being and that participation in fetal transplantation will contribute to the brutalisation of medical personnel. The Polkinghorne Committee denied this charge and argued that material derived from induced abortion carries no moral taint. This argument is not accepted by many in the pro-life movement who would endorse the use of material if and only if it is taken from spontaneous abortions. This, however, would reduce the potential supply considerably, as material from spontaneous abortions is unsatisfactory because it carries a high risk of chromosomal abnormalities and a risk of viral infections. It is also an unsatisfactory source because, owing to the lapse of time between the death of the fetus and its expulsion from the uterus, damage to the tissue may occur.

Neither side in the debate believes that the need for human tissue provides justification for terminating a pregnancy. The point at issue is whether the rights and wrongs of abortion (usually portrayed in terms of competing interests between maternal choice and rights attributed to the developing human being) should be distinguished from arguments concerning the use and potential benefits of fetal tissue research and transplantation.

Robertson (1988) employs an analogy with organs harvested from homicide victims, in order to separate the benefits of fetal transplants from the moral taint of abortion. Pro-lifers certainly view abortion as equivalent to homicide. Yet no one suggests that the benefits derived from the procurement and distribution of organs from murder victims are morally tainted by the mode of death. Moreover, it would be absurd to suggest that surgeons and medical personnel who undertake research on legally obtained cadavers of murder victims are brutalised by their activities. According to this argument it would seem to be acceptable to benefit from what is perceived as an evil without actually applauding the evil.

Another objection is that the potential benefits of fetal tissue transplantation may put pressure on women to conceive and abort in order to produce fetal tissue. One case frequently cited in this context involves the daughter of a man suffering from Alzheimer's disease who petitioned the courts in order to be inseminated with her father's sperm so as to provide him with fetal tissue for a neural transplant (Fine 1988). This, however, was an isolated case and in many respects was an unnecessary request as neural tissue transplants lack antigenicity, thus obviating the need for a close genetic match between donor and recipient.

However, the case that fetal tissue transplantation will encourage induced abortion is strongly advanced, and anti-abortionists argue that if the benefits are widely accepted then the public might become more favourably disposed towards abortion and less likely to support future legislation aimed at reducing the number of induced abortions. It is also argued that a woman in an ambivalent state of mind about an abortion might just be tipped in favour by the utilitarian argument that benefit might accrue from it. Of course, these arguments depend on the respondent sharing the view that further curbs on abortion are morally supportable. Those campaigning for even greater relaxation of abortion laws would hardly endorse this standpoint.

Proponents of fetal tissue research and transplantation maintain that predictions of increased numbers of abortions are speculative and that among the many reasons why women choose abortion the desire to produce fetal tissue for therapeutic purposes is likely to remain insignificant. Yet if we grant a separation between arguments about the rights and wrongs of abortion and the beneficial uses of fetal tissue, supporters of greater relaxation of abortion laws could not appeal to the beneficial use of aborted fetal material as a moral justification for abortion in the first place. On the other hand, for the anti-abortionist there *is* moral complicity. Even if there is no active collaboration in the termination, and maybe not even indirect association that suggests some form of approval, there remains the kind of moral complicity that is bound up with a failure to take steps to prevent that evil. This kind of complicity could be seen to survive the institutional safeguards—for example, avoidance of any connection between the abortion clinic and the transplant surgeons—designed to maintain the separation principle.

A further consideration of the morality of excising organs from brain-dead homicide victims may be relevant at this point in the investigation. It can certainly be argued that there is no evidence to suggest that the growing need for adult cadaver organs has triggered an increase in homicide rates or impeded proposals to reduce mortality rates by means of seat belt regulations or curbs on the use of firearms. It can also be argued that demand for fetal tissue is unlikely to lead to an increase in the number of induced abortions. And just as one can see a reduction in murders and fatal road accidents as morally desirable, while still benefiting from organs harvested from the victims, it would seem that one can maintain a standpoint of either neutrality or moral condemnation of abortion while condoning the benefits derived from the use of fetal remains.

If there is little difference between excising organs from homicide victims and aborted fetuses, then it would seem that one can take either stand in the dispute over the morality of induced abortion and still endorse the benefits of fetal tissue research. It should be noted, however, that endorsement of the separation principle requires that the fetus be regarded as an independent being, akin to an organ donor, not as an unwanted organ. This conclusion has implications for the problem of consent to fetal experimentation. What tips the argument against the appeal to moral taint is that it is potentially too embracing. Any use of human tissue can be linked to some form of evil, as tissue can be put to benefit when taken from the victims of homicide, road accidents, suicide, or the bodies of the poor. Yet there are no moral arguments that link transplant surgeons with murderers, dangerous motorists, and the outcomes of an uncaring and unequal society. Despite strong feelings about the wrongness of abortion there is a long-established tradition of deriving benefit out of wrong: studies of the effect of poverty-induced disease and studies of victims of war and earthquakes have led to benefits, and those who benefit are not the perpetrators of the original tragedy.

Among the threats to the separation principle are practices where the interests in the procurement of fetal material are allowed to influence the timing and method of pregnancy termination. It has been objected that fetal tissue transplantation may involve unnecessary risks to pregnant women as it leads to a situation where the date of the termination is determined by the desire to obtain satisfactory tissue. There is a short answer to this objection: any decision taken with regard to the date of the termination, once termination has been authorised, should be taken with reference to the interests of the mother alone. Any other course would be counter to well-established principles of individual care and the moral rationale underpinning legally performed abortions, namely the overriding interests of the mother.

Attention has been drawn to occasions where there have been modifications in the procedure for termination due to the need for fetal tissue. In an experimental study conducted in Sweden, which involved transplantation of human fetal brain tissue to rats, the method of terminating the pregnancy was altered so as to enhance survival of the tissue. Hence, '[t]o obtain less damaged fetal tissue, the routine vacuum aspiration was slightly modified. After dilation of the cervical canal, but prior to suction, fetal tissue was removed by forceps' (Olsen et al 1987). This kind of practice could have heralded a dangerous step towards shifting moral concern too far in the direction of those who require fetal tissue. There are, however, laws in Sweden that now prevent doctors from varying methods of abortion to suit the convenience of people who want to use fetal tissue.

The fetus and the dead donor rule

Current research proposals are strictly related to the removal of tissues from dead fetuses. It is generally regarded as immoral to extract material from fetuses maintained ex utero, or to remove tissues from fetuses in utero before they are dead. Most guidelines recommend that the fetus to be aborted should be given the same protection as a dying organ donor, stressing that parts should not be removed from, and experiments should not be performed on, a living fetus. But in the face of a strong appeal to the potential benefits that can be derived from experiments on living fetuses, serious inroads into the 'dead donor' rule could be made. Why, it may be argued, should we wait for the fetus to be dead before experimentation is allowed, as it is already doomed because of the impending abortion process? Why wait until its death before permission is sought for its dissection? If abortion is to be allowed, then why not end its life by the removal of vital parts for experimental or transplantation purposes? No doubt there are many benefits to be derived from such a course, but it is not the prime purpose of moral reasoning to advocate *any* course of action insofar as potential benefit can be predicted. An extension of this proposal could quite easily reach sentenced criminals awaiting execution, and children and others suffering from fatal injuries. The potential damage that could thereby be inflicted on the moral status of transplant surgery should be carefully weighed, not to mention widespread moral indignation against harmful experiments on the living, before such actions are tolerated. It is, of course, clearly obvious that any steps to legitimise the removal of organs from the soon-to-be-aborted fetus would undermine the separation principle, on which rests the argument that fetal tissue transplantation can be morally insulated from arguments about the moral taint of abortion.

The fetus as a commodity

The potential use of fetal material has given expression to fears that an entire new bio-industry will be created just to secure and process (utilising sterile and freezing techniques) fetal tissue and organs in order to make them available for commercial use. These fears are understandable, but this problem is not confined to the harvesting of fetal tissue; it is also a concern with regard to adult organ donation and proposals for the further use of human tissue. In recent years a small number of philosophers have argued in favour of a market approach to the procurement of human tissue on the utilitarian premise that the profit incentive would increase the much needed supply. Opponents argue that it is degrading to treat human parts as commodities.

There is very strong resistance to the idea that fetal material should be treated as a marketable commodity. Resistance to the sale of fetal material is partly bound up with beliefs that a fetus, as a developing human being, is 'entitled to respect, according to its status as a living person' (Polkinghorne 1989). As a human being it is not an object that can be bought and sold. Neither fetuses nor children, alive or dead, can be regarded as chattels. This obligation to respect human tissue extends beyond that which is due to a developing human being, as was noted during the public outrage in January 2001 to reports of a scandal in a hospital at Alder Hey where body parts and tissues of deceased infants had been hoarded by doctors without consent of the parents, in violation of Human Tissue Act 1961 Section 1 (2). Further inquiries revealed how thousands of dead children in hospitals across the United Kingdom had been dismembered and stripped of their organs without parental consent. Researchers who appeal to the potential benefits of the commodification of fetal and infant remains are advised to acknowledge the extent of moral respect accorded to fetal and infant remains.

In many respects, however, a fetus is dissimilar to an organ, tumour or discarded tissue, and arguments about the potential sale of human fetuses are not strictly similar to arguments in the current controversy over the potential sale of organs. If the fetus were similar, there would not be such a controversy over induced abortion. There may be objections to the removal of kidneys for commercial transactions but there are no pressure groups in support of the functioning kidney. A fetus is, even if it is unwanted, distinguished by the fact that it possesses the potential to become a member of a human moral community, that it possesses a genetic identity and, when dead, though smaller than a human cadaver, it merits a degree of respect. For this reason the United States Organ Transplant Act 1984 was amended in 1988 to ban 'sales of fetal organs and subparts thereof'. The Health Council of the Netherlands (1994) recommended a principle of non-commercialisation, and in the UK the Polkinghorne Report (1989) went even further than the Peel Report (1972), in its rejection of the profit motive, arguing against 'inducements' such as administrative costs or discounts on fees charged to the woman having an abortion.

One of the problems that has occurred when formulating ethical guidelines for fetal tissue transplantation is that it is not always clear whether writers on the subject view the fetus as an organ, like a kidney or liver, or whether they view it as a (developing) human being. If it is an organ, it can be donated. Moreover, if a case were established in favour of organ sales, so the argument goes, a fetus could be sold. Nolan (1988) was so exasperated by writers who confused fetuses with organs that she wrote a paper entitled 'Genug ist genug: A fetus is not a kidney'. She concluded that use of fetal material should be restricted to abortions performed on ectopic pregnancies, where removal of the fetus is undertaken because its development outside the uterus places the mother in a life-threatening situation. According to Nolan this restriction guarantees that the benefits of fetal tissue transplants are separated from 'moral stigma' attached to abortion.

The problem of consent

Several objections have been raised against the proposal that maternal consent to fetal transplantation is essential. Should a woman who has chosen to abort retain rights regarding the disposal of her fetus? Philosophers and lawyers are divided on this issue. Some argue that there is no basis for seeking the mother's consent to the use of fetal tissue. Others have argued that a decision to terminate a pregnancy is also an effective withdrawal of interest in the disposal of fetal remains. 'Has she not already abdicated responsibility for the fetus by opting for abortion?' asks Harris (1985), who also argues that the fact that the fetus grows inside the body does not provide a basis for the creation of property rights: viruses, tumours and bacteria grow in bodies without endowing the host with property rights over them. Harris's analogy between the fetus and various bacteria and viruses that grow in the body would suggest that the fetus is a form of 'medical waste', equivalent to a placenta following childbirth, or tissue removed during surgery, which can be put to some beneficial use. But public opinion about human tissue is changing and at least one influential inquiry has recommended that consent is sought for *all* uses of human tissue (Health Council of the Netherlands 1994).

Some philosophers and theologians argue that maternal authority extends only to decisions to terminate the pregnancy. In some cases this can even be separated from a decision to kill the fetus. Mason & McCall Smith (1991) point out that: '[t]here is in fact, no certainty that all women seeking a termination of pregnancy also seek the destruction of their fetus—indeed one may wonder whether or not the woman's right to control her pregnancy extends to a right to control the destiny of a "viable" fetus.'

It is important to separate two aspects of abortion: the termination of the pregnancy and the killing of the fetus. These are morally distinct, although in early abortions termination of pregnancy usually involves killing the fetus. Later in pregnancy, however, the fetus could, with medical assistance, survive removal from the uterus. Arguments that support abortion on the grounds that a woman has the right to terminate an unwanted pregnancy may be covered by arguments supporting the first aspect but might not be extended to her wish for the fetus to be dead. For example, several arguments in favour of termination of unwanted pregnancy often refer to one's right not to have one's body employed as a life-support for another being without consent. This argument could not be extended to grant a wish for the other being to be dead. Yet many arguments in favour of abortion do express a desire beyond termination of pregnancy, to the desire not to be a parent in the biological sense. In this case, should the mother's wish for the death of the fetus be respected? The resolution of this problem may well have some bearing on the problem of maternal authority over the disposal of aborted fetal tissue.

If one argues that the mother should give consent to the use of her fetus for experimental or transplantation purposes, it is important to indicate why. Does she give consent because the fetus is hers to donate, because it is part of her body like a kidney or bone marrow donation? Fetal tissue and organs are unlike organs that can be given up from her body; they are the organs of another body that has grown within her body. This distinction has been employed to limit maternal authority over the disposal of fetal material. Thus Ramsey (1975) argued that '[w]hen a parent resolves to destroy her unborn, she abdicates her right to make decisions on the fetus' behalf'. In a similar vein Burtchaell (1989) argued that 'the decision to abort is an act of such violent abandonment of the maternal trust that no further exercise of such responsibility is admissible'. According to Burtchaell there are limits to parental authority, namely that it is constrained by the moral duties of guardianship. Hence '[w]hen a parent resolves to destroy her unborn she has abdicated her office and duty as guardian of her offspring and therefore forfeits her tutelary powers' (Burtchaell 1989). Burtchaell also refers to a letter from former US President, Ronald Reagan, which says that 'the use of any aborted child for these purposes raises the most profound ethical issues, especially because the person who would ordinarily authorize such use—the parent—deliberately renounces parenthood by choosing an abortion' (personal communication to Joseph R Stanton MD, of the Value of Life Committee 1989).

Clearly, the foregoing argument views the aborted fetus as morally equivalent to a cadaver, and the issue turns on views regarding respectful treatment of cadavers. If parts are to be removed from a cadaver then respect for that cadaver requires either prior permission from the deceased (usually in the form of a donor card) or authorisation from a guardian (usually a spouse or parent). Yet the one who has made the decision to destroy the fetus is also the very same person who is likely to be asked to act as guardian of its remains. In this respect the issue of maternal consent is the crucial link between arguments about abortion and proposals for fetal tissue research and transplantation. An analogy here might be with a man who has just murdered his wife being invited to act as executor of her estate. But there are limits to this analogy and it is not clear what moral force it possesses, thus indicating a crucial weakness in the case against maternal consent. Chadwick (1994) argues that it is not a fair analogy because 'the point is that the mother is thought, in cases of lawful abortion, to have the right to consent to the death of the fetus. The murderer is never thought to have such a right. The positions of the mother and the murderer are therefore fundamentally dissimilar.'

The argument about consent can be taken further. If those responsible for the abortion are prohibited from decisions concerning the use of fetal material, then authority over the disposal of the fetus must be withheld from the doctor or any other medical personnel involved in the abortion, as they too are involved in the destruction of the fetus. In any case doctors and hospitals have no grounds for exercising proprietorial rights over the bodies of their former patients. Does this mean that authority should rest with the father? This too raises problems, admittedly of a different kind, as in many abortion decisions the father is unavailable or has already agreed to the abortion. In that case should authority lie with the government or its agents, the courts or coroners? Objections have been raised against this proposal because, by legitimising abortion in the first place, so it is argued, the government forfeits any moral claim to guardianship of the fetus. The consequences of this argument are ambiguous, i.e. that no one has any moral basis for the authorisation of the use of fetal tissue. This, however, is unsatisfactory as it could mean that no one should be allowed to use fetal tissue or that in the absence of any authority free use can be made of fetal tissue.

Conclusion

What should tilt the balance in favour of maternal consent is an understanding of the context and background to the abortion. Abortion is very often a dramatic experience. The morally sensitive nature of the fetus, even when dead, is inescapably linked to the painful nature, for the woman concerned, of the circumstances of the abortion. In this respect there is a strong case for requesting maternal consent. Add to this a recognisable recent development in moral values towards seeking consent for further use of human tissue that was formerly regarded as 'medical waste', it seems that consent should be obtained for any proposed use of human tissue. In cases involving aborted fetal tissue, the Dutch report recommended that tissue can be used unless the woman, having been previously informed that it may be used, makes an objection, whereas in cases of spontaneous abortion it was recommended that her express consent is required (Health Council of the Netherlands 1994). While this proposal rightly regards maternal consent to be essential, it nevertheless draws an implicit and unnecessary distinction between procedures for consent, or objection in the case of a wanted pregnancy, and procedures for consent after abortion in an unwanted pregnancy. If the public benefits derived from the use of fetal tissue are to be separated from any moral stigma associated with voluntary abortion, the way forward is to require express consent for any proposed use of fetal tissue.

ETHICAL ISSUES IN STEM CELL RESEARCH

Introduction

Stem cells are precursors of cells that remain unspecialised and can go on to form a number of different cell types. The ability to isolate human stem cells from the inner mass of embryos and primordial germ cells of fetuses, and the possible differentiation in tissue culture into various other cell types, such as nerve or heart cells, raises dramatic hopes for the treatment of disease. Stem cell research hovers on the border between science fiction and normal science. Arguments for and against this research have transcended scientific debate, whereby opposing sides have adopted extreme political stances. Opponents speak of the commodification of human life in the interests of corporate organisations, while supporters warn of the emergence of an anti-scientific police state, where the search for truth through scientific research is criminalised. The following discussion will avoid either extreme, but will identify the ethical issues, and draw distinctions between different kinds of discourse that have become entangled in the debate.

Benefits of stem cell research

Stem cells intrigue scientists because they have the potential to differentiate into specialised cells such as the heart, muscle, blood or brain, which could, according to scientific predictions, be used to grow neurones for people with Alzheimer's and Parkinson's disease, or repair spinal cord injuries, and be employed in the treatment of diabetes and heart problems. There may also be the prospect of an advance in our understanding and treatment of cancer, and congenital defects and metabolic diseases in young children. New theories of ageing suggest that DNA damage is responsible for ageing, which raises expectations that the replacement of certain stem cells will increase the human lifespan. The possibility of growing tissues for organ replacement offers a solution to the chronic shortage of organs and the controversy over organ sources: if the cells for transplantation were derived from the insertion of the patient's own somatic cell nucleus into a stem cell, the resulting cell line would be compatible with the patient's cells, thus avoiding problems of tissue rejection and the need for anti-rejection drugs.

Although adult stem cells can reproduce themselves they do not—according to the present level of scientific knowledge—offer the same therapeutic potential as embryonic stem cells. So far, stem cells found in adults have limited potential; brain cells cannot make liver cells, whereas stem cells taken from a ball of some 60 cells that form about 6 days after a human egg is fertilised, are thought to be capable of forming every type of tissue in the body.

Stem cell research is parasitic on human embryo research, which is bound up with research and treatment surrounding human fertilisation and assisted reproduction. In this field, too, the predicted benefits are significant, including the enhancement of reproductive interests, prevention of congenital defects, genetic diagnosis, and assistance with studies on early human development.

Opposition to stem cell research

Despite the predicted benefits of stem cell research there is considerable opposition. Obtaining fetal stem cells involves the destruction of a human embryo, which many opponents equate with taking human life. The wider context should also be considered, involving a distrust of science and its close relationship with corporate interests, fears concerning the commodification of life, and the ongoing controversy regarding abortion. These concerns have found political expression in a ban by the German Parliament on the production of embryonic stem cells from January 2002, although research in Germany can be carried out on imported stem cells. There are prohibitions on research in Denmark, Ireland, Austria and Spain. Stem cell research is allowed in the UK, Israel, the Netherlands, Sweden and the USA, although Federal funding in the latter is restricted to surplus embryos after IVF therapy. To date there is no ruling from Belgium, Greece, Italy, Luxembourg, Portugal and Switzerland (Das Parliament 2002).

Alleged linkage with the controversy over abortion

Research on human stem cells involves the destruction of the embryo, which some opponents have equated with destruction of a fetus. Thus much of the argument about stem cell research has closely resembled arguments considered previously, about research on aborted fetuses, where the root objection is against the voluntary termination of pregnancy. These arguments—which we shall address later—focus on the moral status of the developing embryo. Here we encounter notions regarding the absolute sacredness of life that are juxtaposed with predicted utilitarian benefits. With regard to research on fetal tissue, as we have noted, guidelines have been developed in many countries and put into practice, whereby a principle of separation is maintained between the moral and legal issues surrounding abortion and the regulations governing research and use of fetal material.

Current guidelines on stem cell research in Europe and USA attempt to strike an intermediate position between having total respect for the embryo as a person and having no respect for a cluster of cells. This intermediate position gives embryos a higher moral status than a cluster of cells, but not an equal status to infants and adults. But insofar as embryos are morally significant, there is an opportunity to apply the separation principle of organ transplantation ethics—the organs of the dead can be used, but the good arising out of this cannot justify either killing or hastening the death of the donor (Lamb 2000). In the case of aborted fetuses the separation principle insists that, although use of tissue from the dead fetus is morally acceptable, the benefits derived from it cannot justify the decision to terminate the pregnancy. In this way research on aborted fetuses can be morally insulated from arguments on either side of the abortion debate. With regard to stem cell research, some authorities insist that the pursuit of a similar form of moral neutrality may require limiting research to the 'surplus' embryos destined for destruction after IVF therapy.

An in vitro fertilisation programme creates surplus embryos for which there are the following options: destroy them; preserve them for possible further use; or employ them for research. Thus while there are objections to the creation, and hence destruction, of embryos for research it is argued that embryos created for the treatment of infertility—if they are no longer needed—could be employed for research. According to this proposal any complicity with abortion will be avoided, as the objective in the production of embryos in an IVF programme is to enable pregnancy, not to terminate it.

Nevertheless, we must consider objections to this proposal. In doing so we should be aware of the fact that most questions in reproductive ethics focus on the moral status of the human conceptus. Hence those who argue that a fetus or an embryo is a being with certain rights will maintain that the possession of those rights should provide protection against use for scientific research that involves its destruction. This would automatically rule out research on surplus embryos after IVF therapy. It is widely recognised that the scientific ideal of freedom of enquiry is limited by concern for the value and dignity of human beings. In this way the debate over research on fetuses and embryos has focused on their respective moral status.

Several feminist bioethicists have attempted to broaden the discourse on stem cell research in a similar manner to feminist perspectives on abortion. According to Lisa H Harris (2000): 'For feminist scholars and for many women, abortion has never been solely an issue of the moral status and rights of the fetus. Abortion has always been about the contexts and relationships in which pregnancy occurs.' In a similar vein Harris suggests that discourse on stem cell research involves broader issues than concern over the status of the embryo. Drawing an analogy between the feminist approach to abortion and ethical discourse on stem cell research, she supports 'federally funded, scientifically sound embryo research' on the basis of two feminist claims:

> first, that the relationship and contexts of procreation are important
> factors in the ethics of reproductive decision making, and second,

that one may wish to protect fetal interests, yet agree that sometimes the balance of competing interests outweighs that desire. (Harris 2000)

Feminist bioethics redirects the argument beyond the status of the conceptus towards a broader network of responsibilities and commitments, but the autonomy and rights of the procreator are nevertheless limited by awareness of the moral status of the entity concerned. There is no way of escaping this fact. The limits of reproductive autonomy, as well as the limits of ethical research, are bounded by the question of whether one is dealing with subhuman material or an infant. Harris, of course, recognises this when she speaks of the 'wish to protect fetal interests', which presumably are sometimes in conflict with the proposed benefits of scientific research.

Persons and the moral standing of embryos

Arguments about the moral status of the conceptus frequently polarise over the question as to whether the fetus or embryo is a person. In much of the recent bioethics literature, an appeal to the moral status of persons, and hence criteria for personhood, is presented as the central issue. Arguments about abortion have focused on the question of whether the fetus is a person, where the notion of personhood serves as a criterion for moral standing. This has also been the case for categories of non-sentient beings, including patients in a persistent vegetative state, anencephalic neonates, victims of severe neurological disorders, as well as non human animals. In failing to meet criteria for personhood, so it is argued, these beings can be euthanised, treated as means and, subject to autonomous approval of persons responsible for their care, can be employed as research material. In much of bioethical theory, the moral status of persons is determined by their ability to think, interact, and express rational autonomous preferences (Harris 1985, Singer 1979, Singer and Kuhse 1985). Persons are said to possess rights that other living beings do not possess. Critics have drawn attention to the arbitrariness of 'personism', maintaining that criteria for personhood are ontological and have no normative significance (Edwards 2001, Lamb 2001, Teichman 1997).

When ontological criteria for personhood are allowed to supplant moral discourse, we find a situation where either one insists that embryos are persons and are entitled to the moral standing and privileges bestowed on persons, or one argues that they are not persons and can accordingly be regarded as material that can serve some utilitarian objective. Thus, on the one hand, if it is argued that the embryo is a person, or at least has some of the essential features associated with personhood, or the potential to become a person, then the destruction of surplus embryos after IVF therapy is wrong, experiments on embryos are wrong, and the creation of embryos for research is wrong. But if, on the other hand, it is not a person, so the other side argue, then it has no moral standing and there is nothing objectionable about treating it as a means, and under appropriate conditions whereby the donor of the embryo is treated as an autonomous person, it can be created and used for research.

As with the debate on abortion, most people find this simplified dichotomy unsatisfactory. It is obvious that some persons are unfit to be members of a moral community and are justly removed from society, and there are some beings who do not meet criteria for personhood yet are part of a network of care and moral standing. A few stem cells would not meet criteria for personhood but when we consider their remarkable properties they are awesome. If we reflect that this is what we are, that these cells could one day replace us, that in a symbolic sense they represent the future of humanity, this is truly amazing. There is also a sense in which embryonic cells have a similar moral status to the dead. One symbolically represents the past, the other represents the future, although in their immediate state neither are recognised as persons; and we recognise our respect for both by not treating them in a frivolous way.

Tying the debate too exclusively to criteria for personhood fails to capture what, for many people, is the obvious fact that the human embryo evokes moral respect. The USA's National Bioethics Advisory Commission (1999) drew a distinction between human embryos and persons according to a grading criterion whereby 'the embryo merits respect as a form of life, but not at the same level of respect accorded to persons'. While this standpoint correctly recognises the element of respect due to embryos, it nevertheless reveals a peculiar view of moral enquiry as some form of grading exercise, with persons at the summit. What should be recognised is the obvious fact that entities in the world do not possess levels of moral worth that can be measured, but are entitled to the kind of respect accorded in the context in which they are encountered.

It is this notion of respect for the embryo—so difficult to encapsulate once the parameters of moral discourse have been limited to criteria for personhood—which explains the unease expressed in objections to the commodification of human tissue and distrust of the global institutions of medicine and biotechnology. The use of embryos as therapeutic resources or experimental material represents an instrumental view of human life with wide-ranging social implications. However, the acknowledgement that embryos are objects of respect need not support a total prohibition on experiments and research, conducted within ethical parameters, where the objectives are treating diseases and saving lives, which is a means of showing respect for life.

Very often the way forward in ethical argument is to consider the application of established principles to new areas of moral enquiry. Principles governing research on embryos might borrow from principles governing research on animals, where it is recognised that such research may be essential if medical science is to effectively combat certain diseases, and also recognised that researchers have a moral obligation towards animal welfare (Balls et al 1994). Many animal experimenters have taken an intermediate position between a total ban on experiments and complete freedom of enquiry. Thus ethical principles governing animal research have been introduced, such as the three Rs—replacement, reduction, and refinement; that is, experimenters must seek ways in which animals can be replaced; they must find ways to reduce the number of animals used in experiments, and they must refine their experiments so as to minimise harm and destruction. As long as it is not maintained that human embryos are identical to laboratory animals, the analogy may hold insofar as they are beings whose moral standing is at present a matter of dispute.

An intermediate position of this kind could be considered for stem cell research, where it would be recognised that embryos have moral standing, the extent of which remains a matter of dispute, and that their use and destruction must be subject to ethical restrictions. In this way a modified version of the principle of the three Rs would involve asking whether stem cells from human embryos can be *replaced* with adult cells. There are suggestions that this may be possible if, for example, stem cells taken from bone marrow in adults can be developed into any tissue found in the body (Pagan 2002). Likewise it can be asked whether the number of embryos required can be *reduced*, and finally whether experimental techniques can be *refined* in order to minimise harm and maximise respect. As in the case of animal research, these principles do not provide absolute protection, but they do ensure that forms of life that are experimented on in order to bring benefit are nevertheless regarded as a source with moral significance, while debates continue with regard to the *extent* of their moral significance.

Evidence of benefit should weigh up competing interests and be more concrete than appeals to the ideal of open-ended research, or rhetorical appeals to misunderstood scientific pioneers such as Galileo and Giordino Bruno. If we grant scientists the right to enquire into these areas, they in turn have an obligation to provide greater precision regarding their forecasts. In this context it must also be considered that medical scientists have a moral duty to take reasonable steps to improve the human condition, and that stem cell research is justifiable if it can do this.

The accuracy of scientific forecasts of benefit therefore becomes an important moral requirement. In addition, the following ethical issues will have to be addressed.

Maternal consent and risks

If surplus embryos after IVF therapy are to be used then consent should be obtained from the woman who has produced them. This should involve three options: storing them, donating them to another woman, or discarding them. Only in the third case should the option to donate them for research be introduced, together with information that the embryos will be destroyed during the research process.

Although it is sometimes argued that there is no difference between surplus embryos from IVF therapy and 'cells' produced for research (Macklin 2000), from the woman's standpoint there is a significant difference. Ovarian hyperstimulation involves risks of thrombosis, liver or kidney failure and, according to some studies, risks of ovarian cancer. There is risk of pain and injury due to the retrieval procedure, as well as psychological and emotional stress (Baylis, 2000). It is possible that in the near future, with in vitro oocyte maturation, several risks can be eliminated, but this would not include the psychological and emotional effects and discomfort experienced during the retrieval process (Baylis 2000).

These risks may be considered worth taking by a woman who hopes to benefit from a genetically related child, although questions might be raised with regard to her comprehension of the risks when the decision is made in the context of fulfilling a deep-rooted desire for a child. According to one study, out of 52 infertile patients who were receiving ovulation-induction drugs, 79% were willing to accept a suspected possibility of ovarian cancer against the benefits of prospective pregnancy (Rosen et al 1997). If respect for embryos forbids their creation for financial gain, awareness of these risks would certainly reduce the number of volunteers willing to produce embryos for research purposes. Moreover, the battery of medical tests and painful procedures and the requirement to disclose personal medical information, with no control over who receives the donation, would create an even greater disincentive to donate.

The problem of surplus embryos

Guidelines in the USA and Germany appear to recognise a distinction between embryos created for research and those arising as surplus after IVF therapy. In the USA federal funding is only available for research on the latter, with the rationale being that as the surplus embryos are to be discarded anyway, there is no ethical objection to attempts to derive benefit from research conducted on them. How valid is the distinction between embryos created for research and the surplus from IVF therapy? To put the question another way: is the creation of a surplus of embryos that will be used in research any different to the creation of embryos for research? What is a surplus? Is a surplus of embryos necessary?

Cohen (2000) wonders whether embryos are deliberately overproduced in IVF clinics. IVF research, she points out, is largely developed in private medicine where there is less public scrutiny. She argues for greater precision with regard to the notion of 'an excess of embryos', and advocates regulation aimed at reduction in the practice of overproduction. This application of the principle of reduction (mentioned in the discussion of the three Rs) would allay moral concern over the destruction of embryos and reduce risks to women undergoing hyperstimulation.

Linkage with concerns over genetically altered human beings

When approaching new scientific issues, it is important to consider whether they introduce new ethical problems or revise longstanding ones. The prospect of altering the genetic make-up of human beings or creating designer children has fascinated scientists and bioethicists and has created public alarm. There are suggestions that stem cell research may contribute to research on genetically altered human beings. The longevity of embryonic stem cells gives researchers ample time to add or delete DNA, thus the isolation of the embryonic stem cell makes it possible for what is called 'germ line genetic intervention', whereby the nuclear DNA from an infertile woman's egg can be combined with DNA from the female donor's egg to produce a genetically altered germ line cell. In this way the technology associated with assisted reproduction can be combined with the technology for gene transfer, giving rise to the possibility of a genetically altered child. Parens (2000) has drawn attention to this possible convergence of reproduction technology and genetic technology, calling it 'Reprogenetics', which, he concludes, will require the creation of a public institution, isolated from extremists on both sides of the abortion debate, that will contemplate the ethics of reprogenically shaping our children.

Conclusion

From the ethical standpoint the question is whether there are good reasons to permit stem cell research that requires the destruction of human embryos. Weighing up risks and benefits involves finding a balance between well-founded scientific predictions of greater human benefit as against the destruction of an entity that, for many people, is an object of moral significance. There is a further task of weighing up risks and benefits involving the woman who produces the embryos, where it can be argued that there is greater benefit to the woman who produces surplus embryos in the context of attempting to fulfil a desire for a genetically related child. With regard to the status of the embryo it would seem that there is no morally significant distinction between those created for research and the surplus embryos created for reproduction (Macklin 2000). If the embryo is regarded as having a similar moral status to a fetus or an infant, then either source is questionable, but if we recognise that it is like many other life forms we regard as morally significant, then scientists are required to produce overwhelming evidence that the fruits of their research *will*—not may—benefit the many human beings who suffer from the diseases that this research promises to combat. I have argued that the embryo does not have to fulfil ontological criteria for personhood in order to merit moral recognition, and that one way of demonstrating this recognition is to develop principles applied to experiments on other life forms, such as the principle of three Rs, where efforts to replace, reduce or refine the use of embryos are operative.

References

Balls M, Festin, M F U, Flecknell P A 1994 The three Rs: developments in laboratory animal science. Laboratory Animals 28:193–231

Baylis F 2000 Our cells/ourselves: creating human embryos for stem cell research. Women's Health Issues 10:140–145

British Medical Association 1988 Medical ethics: transplantation of fetal material. British Medical Journal 296:1410

Burtchaell J 1989 The use of aborted fetal tissue in research and therapy. In: Burtchaell J (ed) The giving and taking of life: essays ethical. University of Notre Dame Press, Illinois p 155–187

Chadwick R F 1994 Corpses, recycling and therapeutic purposes. In: Lee R, Morgan D (eds) Death rites: law and ethics at the edge of life. Routledge, London p 54–71

Cohen C B 2000 Use of 'excess' human embryos for stem cell research: reinscribing the abortion debate. Women's Health Issues 10:146–151

Coutts M C 1993 Fetal tissue research: scope note 21. Kennedy Institute of Ethics Journal 3:81–101

Department of Heath and Social Security 1972 The use of fetuses and fetal material for research: Report of the Advisory Group (the Peel Report). HMSO, London

Edwards S D 2001 Philosophy of nursing. Palgrave, Basingstoke

Fine A 1988 The ethics of fetal tissue transplants. Hastings Center Report 18(3):5–8

Harris J 1985 The value of life. Routledge, London

Harris L H 2000 Ethics and politics of embryo and stem cell research: protecting women's rights and health. Women's Health Issues 10:121–126

Health Council of the Netherlands: Committee on Human Tissue for Special Purposes 1994 Proper use of human tissue. Health Council of the Netherlands, The Hague

Lamb D 2000 Transplante de orgãos ética. Editora Hucitec, São Paulo

Lamb D 2001 Ética, morte e morte encefálica. Office Editora e Publicidade, São Paulo

Macklin R 2000 Ethics, politics, and human embryo stem cell research. Women's Health Issues 10:111–115

Mason J J, McCall Smith R A 1991 Law and medical ethics, 3rd edn. Butterworths, London

Masstab fur jede Bewertung is und bleibt die Menschenwurde 2002 Das Parliament 52 (18, 03/05):18

National Bioethics Advisory Commission 1999 Ethical issues in human stem cell research. National Bioethics Commission, USA

Nolan K 1988 Genus ist genug: a fetus is not a kidney. Hastings Center Report 18:13–19

Olsen L, Stromberg I, Bygdeman M et al 1987 Human fetal tissues grafted to rodent hosts: structural and functional observations of brain, adrenal and heart tissues in oculo. Experimental Brain Research 67:163–178

Pagan S 2002 Is this the one? New Scientist 26 January p 4–5

Parens E 2000 Embryonic stem cells and the bigger reprogenetic picture. Women's Health Issues 10:116–120

Polkinghorne Committee 1989 Review of the guidance on the research use of fetuses and fetal material (the Polkinghorne Report) HMSO, London

Ramsey P 1975 The ethics of fetal research. Yale University Press, New Haven

Robertson J A 1988 Rights, symbolism and public policy in fetal tissue transplants. Hastings Center Report 18:5–12

Rosen B, Irvine J, Ritvo P et al 1997 The feasibility of assessing women's perceptions of the risks and benefits of fertility drug therapy in relation to ovarian cancer risk. Fertility and Sterility 68:90–94

Singer P 1979 Practical ethics. Cambridge University Press, Cambridge

Singer P, Kuhse H 1985 Should the baby live? The problem of handicapped infants. Gregg, Aldershot

Teichman J 1997 Polemical papers. Ashgate, Aldershot

Chapter **10**

Reproductive technologies and midwifery

Lucy Frith

INTRODUCTION

Reproductive technology is an area of rapid change and expansion. There are new procedures and techniques reported with unnerving regularity and it may seem to the midwife that it is almost impossible to keep up to date. This chapter aims to introduce the most common assisted conception procedures, to outline the role of the law and the relevant legislation in this area and to consider the main ethical dilemmas that have arisen from these scientific developments. Finally, the chapter will focus on areas where reproductive technologies could directly affect midwifery practice. Clearly, when dealing with such a huge area the chapter cannot hope to be exhaustive, but the main points of the debates and controversies will be highlighted and the reader directed to further sources.

ASSISTED REPRODUCTION PROCEDURES

In vitro fertilisation (IVF)

Many people are familiar with the basic notion that IVF involves fertilisation outside the woman's body; the combination of procedures that go to make up an IVF treatment cycle is probably less well known. The treatment begins with the stimulation of the ovarian cycle with superovulatory drugs. This is deemed preferable to the natural cycle for two reasons; first, ovulation can be timed precisely, enabling the retrieval procedure to be scheduled in advance; and second, it produces multifollicular development and a greater number of oocytes can be retrieved. This is desirable 'because pregnancy rates are higher with the transfer of more than one pre-embryo' (American Society for Reproductive Medicine 1998). The degree of superovulation is monitored by oestrogen assays and/or ultrasound scanning (RCOG 1992). The oocytes are then retrieved, most commonly, by the transvaginal ultrasound-guided route. This can be performed under sedation and is preferable to retrieval techniques that need to be performed under general anaesthetic. The sperm and oocytes are then co-incubated for approximately 12–18 hours so that fertilisation can occur. Sometimes embryos are created for IVF using intracytoplasmic sperm injection (ICSI) where a single sperm is injected into an egg. ICSI is used where the male partner's sperm count is low. The process has about the same success rate as conventional IVF, but there are concerns that the resulting children have a higher rate of birth defects. After 24 hours the embryos should have cleaved twice to the four-cell stage and up to two are placed in the uterus transcervically by means of a fine catheter.

Other techniques

The other most common infertility treatment is gamete intrafallopian transfer (GIFT). Eggs are collected in the same way as IVF and then sperm and a maximum of three eggs are transferred together into one or both of the woman's fallopian tubes, replicating the site of natural fertilisation. This does not involve the creation of an embryo outside the body and is only suitable for women whose fallopian tubes are healthy.

Reproductive cloning has been receiving increased attention since the development of cell nuclear replacement (CNR), the process used to create Dolly the sheep, but identical twins could also be created by dividing the developing embryo at an early state. The former process has attracted interest as a means of cloning a specific individual. It has been suggested that CNR could be used instead of donated gametes to ensure that individuals could have a genetically related child (albeit one who was identical to themselves). The latter process could be used by individuals to maximise the chances of a successful pregnancy when they only have one embryo available for implantation. Reproductive cloning using CNR is illegal in the UK but at the time of writing there have been reports of successful pregnancies in humans elsewhere in the world, but these have yet to be verified. Reproductive cloning has been distinguished from therapeutic cloning, which is legal in the UK. Therapeutic cloning uses CNR, but the embryos created are subject to the same restrictions as those used for research (see later) and it would be illegal to implant them. Therapeutic cloning is part of the effort to develop stem cell technology (which is discussed in Chapter 9). For a discussion of issues surrounding therapeutic cloning see DoH (2000).

Finally, it is worth mentioning artificial insemination (AI), where a woman is inseminated artificially with sperm (from her partner or from a donor) either at the cervical opening or into the cervical canal. This simple procedure requires no medical involvement, it is something that one could do at home with the help of a turkey baster (a tool often mentioned in the literature, although there may be other more suitable vehicles!).

REGULATION AND LEGISLATION

Scientific developments in embryology and techniques such as embryo transfer culminated in the birth of the world's first test-tube baby in Britain in 1978. It was recognised that such developments, which concerned the very creation of life itself, had to be debated publicly and the ethical and social dimensions of these techniques assumed increasing importance. The Committee of Inquiry into Human Fertilisation and Embryology (the Warnock Committee) was set up in 1982. The Warnock Committee reported in 1984 and recommended statutory regulation of medically assisted reproduction.

As a result, the Human Fertilisation and Embryology Act 1990 was passed to regulate such procedures as embryo transfer, embryo research, the storage of gametes and embryos, and the use in treatment of donated gametes (eggs and sperm) and of embryos produced outside the body. It was recognised, however, that in such a rapidly changing area it would be impossible to legislate for all future possibilities and developments, and that any legislation might quickly become out of date and hence unworkable in practice. So the Act provided for the creation of a regulatory body, The Human Fertilisation and Embryology Authority (HFEA), to continually revise the provision of services, issue licences to clinics and formulate policy on new developments.

Statutory regulation of medical procedures is by no means uncontroversial, as Kennedy & Grubb (1994) note, 'in general, particular aspects of medical practice are rarely regulated by statute in England. The 1990 Act is a significant exception to this; perhaps reflecting the fine balance between assisting the infertile and the fears of what could flow from the technologies as they are developed'. The USA, for instance, does not have similar all-encompassing legislation, leaving certain questions up to the discretion of individual doctors (American Society for Reproductive Medicine 1998).

The legislative response to the problems of assisted conception can be criticised on the grounds that it limits the clinical freedom of doctors and scientists. It could be argued that a regulatory body is too blunt an instrument to adequately oversee research because as this is an area of such rapid development, there could be delays in research progress while the issues are debated publicly. Against this I would argue that the interests of scientists should not be allowed to override those of society; constant questioning and an appraisal of each new development are imperative to ensure that scientists practise in an ethical way.

The HFEA

The statutory functions of the HFEA are to license and monitor clinics, regulate the storage of gametes and embryos, produce a code of practice as a form of guidance for good practice in clinics, keep a formal register of information relating to donors, treatments and children resulting from treatment, publicise their role and provide information, and keep abreast of new developments in the area with a view to advising the government. 'Underlying all these activities is the HFEA's determination to safeguard the interests of patients, children, doctors, scientists, the wider public and future generations' (HFEA 2002a). The HFEA produces an annual report, annual statistics, information leaflets for patients, and information for clinics and the media, all of which can be found on their web site www.hfea. gov.uk. The HFEA issues licences for clinics that last for 3 years, and clinics are inspected every 3 years with a view to renewing, restricting or revoking their licence. Additional licences have to be sought for embryo research and the use of techniques like preimplantation genetic diagnosis (PGD). Decisions to issue specific licences can be controversial, as happened in 2002 when the HFEA permitted Mr and Mrs Hashmi to use PGD not only to select an embryo that was unaffected by the genetic condition threatening the life of their son, but also to select an embryo that could act as a stem cell donor to provide treatment to save his life. This decision to permit the creation of a so-called 'saviour sibling' was controversial enough on its own, but additional controversy was generated when the HFEA refused permission to another couple, Mr and Mrs Whittaker, to use PGD to select a saviour embryo for their child on the grounds that the condition suffered by their existing child was not genetic in origin (see Chapter 8). The Hashmi decision was successfully challenged in the courts by the Pro-life Alliance and at the time of writing the case has gone to appeal.

Not only does the HFEA monitor scientific developments, it also considers the ethical acceptability of all aspects of assisted conception, 'respond[ing] to public concern about the social and ethical implications of new techniques' (HFEA 1995). One way in which it has done this is by conducting public consultations on controversial and emerging issues. This has included two consultations on sex selection (HFEA 1993, HFEA 2002b), donated ovarian tissue (HFEA 1994b), (with the Human Genetics Commission (HGC)) preimplantation genetic diagnosis (HFEA & HGC 2001), and the modernisation of regulation and new fee strategy (HFEA 2002c). Consultation documents have been produced that set out the issue to be considered, producing an overview of the main arguments (as perceived by the HFEA) and an invitation for public response from both individuals and professional bodies. Public consultation appears to facilitate openness, transparency, political inclusion and responsible citizenship. However, the response rate to public consultations is sometimes disappointing, and those run by the HFEA have been no exception (for instance, the 1993 sex-selection public consultation document only produced approximately 200 replies from 2000 documents sent out, while the donated ovarian tissue document produced 25 000 requests for copies and some 9000 replies). Clearly, the general public have yet to feel involved in these decisions and although the response rate to the donated ovarian tissue document was encouraging, it still provoked a response from a relatively small proportion of the general public.

Who is the parent?

The separation of sex and procreation requires us to think more carefully about how to answer the question 'what is a parent?'. In the past, this question was mainly concerned with recognising parents by adoption and the value of the role of the 'social' parent as opposed to the 'natural', 'biological' or 'genetic' parent. Now it is possible, for instance, for a woman to be the biological mother of a child to whom she is not genetically related, or for her to be genetically related to a child who is borne by another woman. The need for greater legal clarity was recognised by the Human Fertilisation and Embryology Act 1990, which laid out how parentage was to be determined for legal purposes.

The father: the husband of the woman undergoing such treatment is treated as the father of the resulting child, unless, 'it is shown that he did not consent to the placing in her of the embryo or the sperm and eggs or to her insemination (as the case may be)' (s28(2)(b)). This provision also extends to a couple who are not married, but receive the treatment services 'together' (s28(3)). Thus the donor is, except in very rare circumstances (see Kennedy & Grubb 1994), protected from becoming the legal father of any child born of his sperm. The provisions of the Act were severely tested in 2002/2003, when it was revealed that sperm from one couple (Mr and Mrs B) was mistakenly used to fertilise eggs from another couple (Mr and Mrs A) and twins were born as a result to Mr and Mrs A. Although children of couples who are married are presumed to be children of that marriage, the court decided that Mr B was the legal father of the children because Mr A had not consented to having his wife's eggs fertilised by another man's sperm. However, as Mr B was not married to Mrs A he was considered for legal purposes like any other unmarried father with no parental rights (unless this is given to him by either the mother or courts). Mr A will have to adopt the twins to become their legal father.

The mother: section 27(1) of the 1990 Act stipulates that the mother of the resulting child is '[t]he woman who is carrying or has carried a child as a result of the placing in her of an embryo or of sperm and eggs, and no other woman, is to be treated as the mother of the child.' Thus it is the gestational function that determines legal motherhood, not the genetic relationship (i.e. if the woman receives a donated egg it is she, not the egg donor, who is deemed to be the mother).

Section 30 of the 1990 Act provides for maternal transfer of parental responsibility (Parental Orders Regulations 1994). This brought into effect new legal instruments called 'parental orders' for use in the case of surrogacy. If a child is born to a surrogate mother then parental orders will allow the transfer of legal parental responsibility from the surrogate parent to the commissioning couple without the need for full adoption procedures. These orders can only be granted when the child is genetically related to at least one of the commissioning couple, who must apply within 6 months of the child's birth; the commissioning couple must be over the age of 18 at the time of making the application, the child must be living with them and they must be domiciled in the UK; and the surrogate (and her husband, if she is married) must have consented no earlier than 6 weeks after the birth. (For more detailed information see, Kennedy & Grubb 1994.)

ETHICAL DILEMMAS

In a chapter of this size it is impossible to do justice to the range of ethical dilemmas that have arisen from the development of artificial reproductive technologies (ART). Hence, I want to concentrate on the main dilemmas that have exercised the policy makers when formulating the 1990 Act and those policy problems that have emerged since the passage of the legislation. I shall first consider the main ethical concerns that preceded the 1990 Act.

Prior to the 1990 Act there was considerable ethical debate about the acceptability of ART themselves. The Warnock Report (1984) characterised these as: 'opposition based on the fundamental principles ... of IVF ... that this practice represents a deviation from normal intercourse and that the unitive and procreative aspects of sexual intercourse should not be separated.' The Report concluded that this view should not be allowed to dictate policy because it was a matter of individual conscience: 'There will be those who will not wish to receive this form of treatment nor participate in its practice, but we would not rely on those arguments for the formulation of public policy.' The fundamental principles that lie behind ART were thereby publicly accepted and the debate over whether to have such ART, in any form, were superseded and replaced with concerns about the type of regulation and how best to ensure that progress in ART proceeds ethically and responsibly.

Using human embryos

The Warnock Committee also extensively debated the use, storage and research protocols concerning embryos. Embryo research was an integral part of the scientific development of IVF and, in enabling embryos to be created outside the body, it has opened up a whole area of debate over the moral status of the embryo (Dyson & Harris 1990, Singer et al 1990). This debate has continued with the development of stem cell research (see Chapter 9). The question is how to regard embryos in a moral sense; that is, some decision needs to be made as to what kind of entity they are, so that embryos can be treated in a morally appropriate way.

At one end of the spectrum, there are those who claim that as the embryo is a human *being* it should be accorded full moral status and therefore be treated the same as any other human being, child or adult. Accordingly, the embryo has a right to life and this must be respected. At the other end, there are those who contend that only human *persons* should be the recipients of moral status. Since person-hood means a self-conscious, thinking, feeling being, the embryo is not a person, it is simply a collection of cells and therefore has no right to life. There have been extensive philosophical debates over these issues and, as illustrated by the abortion debate, very little consensus has been reached (see Hursthouse 1987).

The Warnock Report (1984) framed the question in terms of 'how is it right to treat the human embryo' and concluded that 'the embryo of the human species should be afforded some protection in law'. In effect the middle ground was adopted, not affording the embryo rights on a par with an adult, but not equating the embryo with a morally insignificant clump of cells. The 1990 Act reflected this position and states:

> a licence cannot authorise—keeping or using an embryo after the appearance of the primitive streak ... the primitive streak is to be taken to have appeared in an embryo not later than the end of the period of 14 days beginning with the day when the gametes are mixed. (s3(3) & (4))

This 14-day cut off point has attracted much criticism on the grounds that it is an arbitrary point of demarcation. Warnock (1985) has responded to this criticism by arguing that 'the point was not however the exact number of days chosen, but the absolute neces-sity for there being a limit set on the use of embryos'. Whether or not the 14-day cut off is arbitrary, precise research guidelines, enshrined in legislation, have been established for monitoring by the HFEA (see HFEA 1994a). An amendment was made to the 1990 Act in 2000, extending the reasons for using embryos in research to take advantage of stem cell technology. The amendment came into force in January 2001 and the HFEA's role changed accordingly (see HFEA 2002a).

The creation and use of embryos has given rise to moral difficul-ties for many people and was arguably one of the main reasons why it was thought necessary to regulate ART. Those ART that do not involve the creation of embryos outside the body such as GIFT or AI do not fall under the 1990 Act and are not licensed by HFEA (unless donor gametes are used and/or the procedures take place in licensed clinics). Nonetheless, the HFEA does offer advice on GIFT and has surveyed GIFT clinics (see web site www.hfea.gov.uk).

Access to ART

There has been increasing public and professional concern over the issue of who should have access to ART. Should, for instance, treatment be given to single women; non-heterosexual couples; individuals with a history of crime, mental illness, disability or serious health problems like HIV infection; or post-menopausal women and elderly men? The concerns here are often expressed in the form, 'who is fit to be a good parent?' The HFEA (2001) Code of Practice does not lay down any precise guidelines as to who should or should not receive infertility treatment. However, the well-being of the future children is held to be the paramount consideration. Section 13(5) of the 1990 Act states that:

> A woman shall not be provided with treatment services unless account has been taken of the welfare of any child who may be born as a result of the treatment (including the need of that child for a father), and of any other child who may be affected by the birth.

This suggests that access to infertility treatment should only be denied on the grounds that the future welfare of the resulting child appears to be in jeopardy. Interpreting this section is left to individual centres and practitioners. The HFEA Code of Practice (2001) reminds clinics that no category of woman is excluded from treatment by the 1990 Act; it recommends that centres should have clear written procedures to follow when assessing the future welfare of the child and reminds clinics of the 'importance of a stable and supportive environment for any child born as a result of treatment'. As well as considering the welfare of the future child, consideration, arguably equal consideration, has to be given to existing children. The HFEA (2001) suggests that this includes any other children that a woman has or who are part of her family or living with her.

Single women and lesbian couples would appear at first sight to be excluded from treatment by section 13(5), but this is not the case as the Act only requires that account be taken of the need of the child for a father. The HFEA (2001) suggest that 'where the child will have no legal father ... centres should consider particularly whether there is anyone else ... willing and able to share responsibility for meeting those needs.' This is a relatively progressive provision. Many countries (e.g. France) restrict access to married or stable heterosexual couples.

Another focus of concern has been the issue of whether postmenopausal women should receive infertility treatment. There have been various cases drawn to the attention of the public by the media, most notably the clinic in Italy that treated a 62-year-old woman, believed to be the oldest such mother. In April 1995 a 51-year-old woman gave birth to a daughter after receiving a donor egg. She had lied about her age so that she would be accepted for treatment, telling the clinic she was 47. Should these women have received infertility treatment?

In answering this question, the starting point must be the welfare of the future child, but it is not self-evidently harmful for a child to have parents who are older than normal, and it is not even clear what the normal age for childbearing/rearing is. The Family Policy Studies Centre (1995), in a report examining the birth rate, stated that more women are delaying having children until their late 30s and early 40s. The normal age to have children appears to be slowly rising. Thus it seems to be almost impossible to determine what is the normal age for childbearing in a society where changing social circumstances and improvements in health can shift that point. Clearly, in considering the acceptability of treatment for older women, it is a matter of degree: we might, for instance, think that 60 is too old but 50 is just acceptable. This creates the problem of how we are to justify these two different limits in policy terms, as any decision has to be shown to be both justifiable and equitable.

Clinics have to deal with two kinds of scenario: women who require egg donation (for IVF) and those women who can use their own eggs. The women who require egg donation are not necessarily older women. They might have a high risk of transmitting a serious genetic condition or they may have undergone a premature menopause. However, if a woman is post-menopausal she will require egg donation in order to conceive. It is argued that the menopause could be used as a cut off point for those seeking ART. If the woman has reached the menopause then her fertile time is over (biologically) and this would provide an objective, testable point that was not subject to the individual practitioner's interpretation and judgement. But such a test would exclude women, sometimes in their 20s, who have had their menopause very early, which seems perverse as they are nowhere near the upper age limit that the 'menopause test' seeks to define. One solution would be to use the average age at menopause rather than the actual age at menopause to mark the upper age limit for treatment. This, however, seems equally arbitrary and does not address the problem of what 'normal' should mean in terms of age.

Moreover, it has been argued that 'age related decline in fecundity is associated with the age of the oocytes rather than the age of the uterus' (Abdalla et al 1993). Thus women over 40, although they may have not yet reached menopause, may wish to have donor eggs provided to minimise the risk of miscarriage or conditions such as Down's syndrome. Thus approaching the menopause ceases to be an important cut-off point in terms of the physical welfare of the future child when donor eggs are used (the HFEA (2001) policy is that egg donors must be under 35 save in exceptional circumstances). Again, the problem comes back to making the judgement of whether to treat on the basis of an individual's age, rather than a biologically determined point.

There is also the issue of scarce resources. Although this is a practical consideration, allocation is frequently based on similar concerns about who the best parents will be. Even if we accept in principle that there is nothing inherently wrong with providing treatment for 'older women', due to the shortage of donor eggs many have argued that younger women should be given priority. The Lister Hospital, which treated the 51-year-old in 1995, said that they had 600 women waiting for matched eggs and their main concern was that reports of older women giving birth would put off prospective egg donors. Further, with limited resources provided for infertility treatment within the NHS (ISSUE 1993), decisions will again have to be made on which individual is to be treated.

However, to assert that younger women should be given priority either in terms of treatment or donated eggs, is once again to highlight age as the most significant factor. If there is nothing inherently wrong with being an older mother, age should not be used when allocating resources. If there is something wrong with being an older mother we must devise guidelines that propose a suitable age limit for treatment and that explain why age is significant. A precise age limit is always going to be problematic, but 50 seems to be the working limit of many centres. The HFEA (2001) only requires centres to consider individuals' 'likely and future ability to look after or provide for a child's needs'. If the principle driving the need for an age limit is the capability of an individual to provide future care, account should not be taken of *age* at the time of treatment but *life expectancy* at that time. Someone who is 50 and in good health at the time of treatment may have a better life expectancy than someone who is 30 but whose overall health is poor.

The HFEA (2001) recognises the complexities of making decisions about who should gain access to treatment, and for this reason its guidance is deliberately vague, suggesting only that the needs of the future child must be prominent in any decision made. It is, however, important that individual clinics and practitioners can justify any decisions that they make to exclude individuals from treatment. Some clinics have ethics committees that help them to form policies, although these are often not much more detailed than the HFEA Code of Practice. One of the advantages of having some kind of policy is that it lends a certain amount of transparency to decision-making, and may protect the clinic or individual practitioner from claims of injustice made by disappointed individuals during judicial review.

Disclosure of genetic identity

In 2002, the Department of Health ran its own public consultation on whether the 1990 Act should be amended to grant children created using donated gametes access to additional information about the gamete donor. Children over the age of 18 do have the right under the 1990 Act to gain non-identifying information about the gamete donor from the HFEA under section 31, but the information held by the HFEA is limited (DoH 2001 section 1.27). Moreover, donors are guaranteed anonymity under the 1990 Act.

The consultation seems to have arisen as a result of a combination of events. First, with the completion of the human genome project, genetic information appears to be increasingly important in decisions about medical treatment and prognosis. It could be said that individuals who do not have access to their genetic heritage are at a disadvantage, and if it is possible to reverse this disadvantage by providing the information then, arguably, this should be done. Second, children born as a result of donor gametes have become increasingly vocal about their need to be able to locate themselves within a genetic history. Analogies have been made with adoption and the change in the law that permitted adopted children to learn about the identity of their genetic parents. It is argued that if there was a legitimate need for adopted children to have this information, there is an equally legitimate need for children of gamete donation to have this information. Third, with the implementation of the Human Rights Act 1998, article 8—respect for private and family life—could be used to gain access to information about donors. Indeed in *Gaskin v United Kingdom* [1990] the European Court of Human Rights held that article 8 did indeed serve the purpose of giving individuals a right to establish their genetic identity.

At the time of writing the results of the consultation have not been published, but there are good arguments to support the view that greater access should be granted to identifying information (see Frith 2001).

This section has not covered all the ethical dilemmas created by ART. The development of such technologies has forced us to think about our rights to reproduce, who should reproduce, in what if any circumstances to offer preimplantation genetic screening or diagnosis as part of IVF treatment and what constitutes parental relationships to name a few. These are all questions that are important independently of ART, but ART have posed them with an urgency that has not existed before. It is also worth noting that these discussions have implications for general considerations of parental suitability and so on, and conclusions reached for ART situations can illuminate other areas of such concern.

MIDWIFERY AND REPRODUCTIVE TECHNOLOGIES

Midwives will not be the professionals actively involved in the process of ART. This might lead them to suppose that this subject has no relevance to their profession. However, there are two reasons why a consideration of ART is of use to the midwife. First, midwives, as members of a profession concerned with women and childbirth, should have a general interest in all related areas so that they can take part in public debate on the issues and be able to offer appropriate advice to women in their care. Second, pregnancies and births that result from ART have to be managed and it is here that the midwife could become involved. The number of births resulting from ART in the UK is still relatively small, around 6300 are reported in the provisional HFEA figures for the period ending 2001 (HFEA 2002a). This is, however, twice as many live births as were reported in 1995 for the first edition of this collection (HFEA 1995). The number of individuals being treated continues to rise, as do the success rates, including for women over the age of 38 (HFEA 2002a).

Confidentiality

Midwives are bound by the duty of maintaining confidentiality for all their patients, but for those patients who have received ART there are additional provisions set out in the 1990 Act and the Human

Fertilisation and Embryology (Disclosure of Information) Act 1992. The two main concerns of the 1990 Act were to make sure that children born as a result of ART did not find out inadvertently that they were conceived in this way, and to protect the anonymity of donors.

Those involved in the care of a woman who has conceived as a result of ART have no automatic right to be informed of the circumstances surrounding the conception and the woman is under no obligation to tell her carers, although it is becoming increasingly difficult for individuals to gain access to treatment without agreeing to allow their GPs to be informed. Information can be disclosed, but only with the consent of the person to whom the information relates, and this is subject to clear controls and safeguards. Before the treatment centre discloses any information, reasonable steps must be taken to explain the implications of the disclosure and consent must be obtained in writing. A woman therefore has full control over the information the obstetric team receives. The only exception to this is in the case of an emergency, but if it is practicable to obtain consent for disclosure and this is refused then information must not be disclosed. Once the information has been disclosed it is no longer covered by the 1990 Act, but the common law on confidentiality still applies (HFEA 2001).

These confidentiality provisions affect midwives in two ways. First, as the information regarding infertility treatment is covered by a specific statute, any disclosure must be sanctioned by the person to whom the information relates. It is not accessible under the general provision that professionals involved in a patient's care can have access to that patient's information. Thus the information that midwives might receive could be very limited and they would be unable to attain more even if they felt it was in the patient's best interests. To illustrate this point consider the following hypothetical situation. The midwife might have been told that this is an ART pregnancy by the woman, who has authorised the disclosure of information relating to the drug protocols used in the superovulatory treatment. The midwife becomes concerned about the woman's husband who seems depressed and unwilling to provide any support to his wife. The midwife wonders if the cause of his depression is that he is not the genetic father of the baby. The midwife would like to know if this assessment is correct in order to recommend appropriate counselling for the couple. The woman is very distressed but refuses the midwife's attempts to talk about the situation. However, the midwife cannot find out if the woman has received donor sperm without asking her for authorisation, and is reluctant to do this due to the woman's distress, despite thinking it would be in the patient's best interests to provide this information. Thus this confidentiality provision removes from the midwife a measure of clinical autonomy, as it is left to the client to decide what information should be shared.

Second, as stated, once disclosure has taken place it is no longer covered by the Act. The HFEA (2001) advises that '[c]entres should as far as possible ensure that those receiving information record details of treatment services only on the medical record of the person seeking treatment and not on that of any resulting child.' This is to prevent a child learning, 'in an inappropriate way that they were born as a result of treatment services'(HFEA 2001). So although not under the jurisdiction of the Act, the midwife should be aware of the spirit of the provisions and aim to protect the child from an inadvertent discovery.

The pregnancy

In the management of an ART pregnancy there is the possibility of certain problems arising (which I shall cover next) of which the midwife should be aware. This is not to say that all ART pregnancies will be problematic, but simply that there are some potential pitfalls and if the midwife is sensitive to the possibility then this could provide a better basis for care and support for the woman.

There has been considerable dispute over the contention that all ART pregnancies are necessarily high risk. The HFEA's overall attitude (that is reflected in the confidentiality provisions) is that there is no reason why those managing the birth should be aware of the circumstances of the pregnancy. This assumes there are no particular risks associated with such conceptions. If there are any risks, it could be argued that these are secondary to the treatment; that is, older women and multiple births, and these will be apparent to the midwife without any specific disclosure. In contrast, it has been argued that a 'history of infertility, and particularly a pregnancy resulting from assisted conception should be regarded as a high risk factor in pregnancy' (McFaul et al 1993).

It is beyond the bounds of this chapter to attempt to come to a firm conclusion about which of these risk assessments is correct. It is relevant to simply highlight the *possible* risks that the woman may be subject to, recognising that not all women will be at any significant risk. The ethical implications of these risk assessments will also be considered. For instance, if ART are deemed to produce very high risk pregnancies with little hope of good outcomes, this could tell against the ethical acceptability of ART. I shall consider the issues raised by each stage of pregnancy.

The overall success rate for IVF treatments is around 25% (HFEA 2002a) and it is often noted that this is about the same as the success rate for natural conception. Nonetheless, assisted conception treatment is often stressful and fraught with uncertainty and the experience could affect the attitude of the woman and her general well-being throughout the pregnancy. Individuals receiving assisted conception treatment may have been infertile for several years and even if a pregnancy takes place there is still the possibility of miscarriage. Most women undergo a number of treatment cycles before pregnancy is achieved and this contributes to the stress and strain on the couple. It has been argued that the success rate for IVF suggests that it should be viewed not as a therapeutic procedure but rather as an area of research (Rowland 1993, Spallone 1989). This raises the ethical issue of whether it is justifiable to offer ART to women as a therapeutic procedure if it is more accurate to say they are taking part in a research project. In order to answer this question it is necessary to come to a decision about acceptable levels of success. When is a success rate so low that the technique is still at the research stage? It could also be argued that if ART are still at the research stage then midwives are also unknowingly involved in a research project. This could compromise their professional autonomy as they are not being given the choice as to whether they wish to participate, and they may feel uneasy about their complicity in research dressed up as treatment.

In addition to the stresses inherent in ART, the cause of the infertility may also make the woman more vulnerable to miscarriage during the pregnancy (see Joels & Wardle 1994a) and although all these elements may not be recorded on the patient's notes, they must be borne in mind. Thus understanding and an awareness of such factors can help form the basis for the kind of support the woman needs. Support requirements will be different for every woman and by getting to know her and by the amount of information she chooses to disclose, individual requirements can be gauged.

There are also risks to the woman in undergoing ART, for instance the danger of ovarian hyperstimulation syndrome, which 'is a major complication of ovulation induction … The most severe forms can be life threatening' (Tiitinen et al 1995). There have also been speculative articles that suggest repeated superovulation could be associated with an increase in ovarian carcinoma and this 'is being kept under review' (RCOG 1992). As ART have a relatively short history it is still too early to evaluate the full extent of the risks, including to the future child. These are concerns that will affect other health carers more directly than midwives, but are still concerns of which midwives should be aware.

To turn now to the pregnancy itself, there are two factors that often put the ART pregnancy automatically into a high risk category; first, the women are more likely to be elderly primigravidae—the average age for ART was 34 years of age (HFEA 1994a); and second, they are more likely to be multiple pregnancies. The multiple birth rate was 31.4% for ART compared with 1.25% in the overall population (HFEA 1994a). Both these factors increase the risk of complications throughout the pregnancy.

Bound up with the issues of the risk status of the pregnancy are the possible effects on the provision of neonatal intensive care. One study found that the incidence of preterm births was higher among those who had received ART:

> The high rate of spontaneous preterm labour is in part the result of a high incidence of multiple pregnancy. It may also reflect the effect of ovarian hyperstimulation which results in the uterine environment being exposed to supra-physiological levels of sex steroids at the time of implantation. (McFaul et al 1993)

Thus a higher demand for neonatal care may be apparent in hospitals that provide ART and the planning of maternity services must take into account the demands such pregnancies might make (see Chapter 7).

As Page (1995) states, an important goal of midwifery is to prepare the woman for parenthood and an ART pregnancy could present distinctive demands in this area that need to be ascertained in consultation with the mother. Once birth has taken place, the adjustment to motherhood may be harder to make after such a pregnancy. 'She is more likely than usual to require support and there is evidence that post-partum depression is more common in women whose pregnancies have resulted from assisted conception' (Joels & Wardle 1994b). However, it has been argued that couples who conceive in this way are more prepared for parenthood, and one study argued that the quality of parenting in families with a child conceived by ART is superior to that of families who have naturally conceived children (Golombok et al 1993). The implications of this study are far from clear, but I think it would be fair to say that as all children conceived by ART are very much wanted, this bodes well for the quality of parenthood they will receive.

Finally, it is worth noting that frequently a child born as a result of ART may not be genetically related to one or both of the parents.

How this affects the bonds between children and parents is not yet
well researched, but it is imperative to be aware of this situation and
comments like 'she really looks like her dad' may be very hurtful
when the genetic father is unknown to the couple because donor
sperm has been used.

In summary, ART pregnancies are often very fraught and stressful events for the couple and midwives needs to be sensitive to the
distinctive needs of such a couple. By being aware of the wider
issues and problems raised by ART they can provide appropriate
and skilful care for these women.

CONCLUSION

This chapter has attempted to give a broad overview of the kind of
ethical issues raised by ART. It has also tried to illustrate the distinctive problems that managing these pregnancies might create for
the midwife. It is crucial that midwives follow the debates over ART
so that as individuals and through their professional bodies they can
ensure that these technologies proceed in a way that is beneficial and
not harmful to the women who receive them.

References

Abdalla et al 1993 Age, pregnancy and miscarriage: uterine versus ovarian
    factors. Human Reproduction. 8(9):1512–1517
American Society for Reproductive Medicine 1998 Ethical considerations of
    assisted reproductive technologies. Fertility and Sterility Supplement 3:4
Department of Health 2000 Stem cell research: medical progress with
    responsibility. Department of Health, London
Department of Health 2001 Donor information consultation: providing information
    about sperm, egg and embryo donors. Department of Health, London
Dyson A, Harris J 1990 Experiments on embryos. Routledge, London
Family Policy Studies Centre 1995 Bulletin. Family Policy Studies Centre, London
Frith L 2001 Gamete donation and anonymity: the ethical and legal debate.
    Human Reproduction 16:818–824
Gaskin v United Kingdom [1990] 1 FLR 167
Golombok et al 1993 The quality of parenting in families created by new
    reproductive technologies. Journal of Psychosomatic Obstetrics and
    Gynaecology 14:17–22
Human Fertilisation and Embryology Act 1990 HMSO, London
Human Fertilisation and Embryology (Disclosure of Information) Act 1992
    HMSO, London
Human Fertilisation and Embryology Authority (HFEA) 1993 Sex selection:
    public consultation document. HFEA, London
Human Fertilisation and Embryology Authority (HFEA) 1994a Third annual
    report. HFEA, London

Human Fertilisation and Embryology Authority (HFEA) 1994b Donated ovarian tissue in embryo research and assisted conception public consultation document. HFEA, London

Human Fertilisation and Embryology Authority (HFEA) 1995 Fourth annual report. HFEA, London

Human Fertilisation and Embryology Authority (HFEA) 2001 Code of practice, 5th edn. HFEA, London

Human Fertilisation and Embryology Authority (HFEA) 2002a Eleventh annual report and accounts 2002. HFEA, London

Human Fertilisation and Embryology Authority (HFEA) 2002b Sex selection: choice and responsibility in human reproduction. HFEA, London

Human Fertilisation and Embryology Authority (HFEA) 2002c Consultation on modernisation of regulation and new fee strategy. HFEA, London

Human Fertilisation and Embryology Authority & Human Genetics Commission (HFEA & HGC) 2001 Consultation on preimplanation genetic diagnosis. HFEA, London

Hursthouse R 1987 Beginning lives. Blackwell, Oxford

ISSUE 1993 Infertility: the real costs. The National Fertility Association, Birmingham

Joels L, Wardle P 1994a Causes and treatment of infertility. British Journal of Midwifery 2(9):423–429

Joels L, Wardle P 1994b Assisted conception and the midwife. British Journal of Midwifery 2(9):429–435

Kennedy I, Grubb A 1994 Medical law: text with materials. Butterworths, London

McFaul PB, Patel N, Mills J 1993 An audit of obstetric outcome of 148 consecutive pregnancies from assisted conception: implications for neonatal services. British Journal of Obstetrics and Gynaecology 100:820–825

Page L 1995 Putting principles into practice. In: Page L (ed) Effective group practice in midwifery. Blackwell Science, Oxford

Report of the Committee of Inquiry into fertilisation and embryology (the Warnock Report) 1984 Cmnd 9314. HMSO, London

Rowland R 1992 Living laboratories: women and reproductive technologies. Cedar, London

Royal College of Obstetricians and Gynaecologists (RCOG) 1992 Infertility: guidelines for practice. RCOG Press, London

Singer P et al 1990 Embryo experimentation. Cambridge University Press, Cambridge

Spallone P 1989 Beyond conception: the new politics of reproduction. Macmillan Education, Basingstoke

Tiitinen et al 1995 The effect of cryopreservation in prevention of ovarian hyperstimulation syndrome. British Journal of Obstetrics and Gynaecology 102:326–330

Warnock M 1985 A question of life. Blackwell, Oxford

Chapter **11**

Midwifery and homeopathy
Martien Brands

A 'HOME PERSPECTIVE': THE DUTCH EXPERIENCE

Although homeopathy is practised worldwide, the Netherlands provides a good example of the use of homeopathy in obstetrics. Within the western world, obstetrics in the Netherlands is in the unique position of having 30% of births being home births (Prismant 2000), mostly under the guidance of a midwife (of which some are males). The combination of the respect of some Dutch obstetrics teachers for birth as a natural physiological event and the high level of education of obstetricians has contributed to a situation in which the midwife is considered the lead professional in the guidance of delivery.

Anna Reynvaan, a midwife, was a pioneer in the development of education for obstetricians where medical knowledge had the same importance as developing a sharp observation of the birth process. Knowledge and observation give the Dutch obstetrician the competence to act independently, within the professional limits as formulated in the Obstetrical List of Indications. This is an inventory of the interventions midwives are entitled to practise and gives the indications for referral to an obstetrician or the general practitioner. They constitute a 'framework of competence' (Prismant 1998) for the Dutch obstetrician with clear boundaries with regard to the other professionals in this domain of medical practice and health care.

Knowledge and observation are also the twin pillars supporting reliable homeopathic diagnostics. As specialists in observation of pregnancy and labour, midwives can benefit from the application of homeopathy within the existing framework of professional action, leading to the enhanced effectiveness of interventions. This means that midwifery can continue to be practised as it is, with the addition of homeopathic remedies. A good example is the competent guidance of the process of delivery in cases where the labour is problematic due to physiological disturbances. Naturally, difficulties in labour due to problems such as breech presentation of the child continue to indicate the need for specialist obstetrical care.

Accordingly, many planned home births do not need to be interrupted by a referral to a hospital. Statistics from the Amsterdam Maternity Centre suggest that about 30% of all pregnant women finally deliver at home, out of the 45% who initially choose a homebirth, meaning that in these cases there were no medical or social indications for hospital delivery (Prismant 2000). This implies that 15% of pregnant women are unable to have a home birth due to physiological occurrences during the delivery. At a time when there is increasing demand on health care resources, a rise in the number of home births could make existing hospital services more readily available for those who really need them, while simultaneously empowering healthier pregnant women by the use of homeopathic remedies. In countries other than the Netherlands, home birth may also be considered a safer option with the addition of homeopathic remedies. Extensive experience in the UK and the US suggests that homeopathic remedies in obstetrics are a reliable patient-oriented addition to the existing practice (Castro 1992, Zaren 1989).

In recent years there has been a significant increase in the amount of both clinical and basic research into the effectiveness and efficacy of homeopathy (Kleijnen et al 1991, Linde et al 1997). The results suggest that using homeopathic remedies alongside general medical knowledge now warrants serious consideration. There is particular evidence of good results in pregnancy and labour (Beal 1998), and many case reports have been documented.

This chapter seeks to document a part of this experience, with thanks to all those midwives who have contributed to the current database with careful registration of their patients.

EVIDENCE AND PROFESSIONAL AUTONOMY

To acquire a clear picture of the ethical issues around the use of homeopathy, some specific observations must be made. This form of medicine has, despite existing for two centuries, met with fierce resistance from traditional allopathic medicine, which has acquired the dominant position in western countries. It is not only the legitimacy of homeopathy that has been questioned, however, herbal medicine, Chinese medicine and ayurvedic medicine have all met with scepticism. Although they are globally practised on a large scale, they have never acquired the status of allopathic medicine in the western world because of some anthropological divergences from basic ideas in western science. The perception of disease as a local and material process originated in the 18th and 19th centuries, and this concept implied a different approach to other forms of medicine. The latter advocated a more systemic understanding of disease, where disease of a single organ is considered to be a manifestation of imbalance in the organism as a whole. Therapy, according to this approach, therefore addresses this whole rather than seeking to eliminate a disturbance arising from one organ or one external microorganism.

After decades of success, it has become apparent that interactions and side-effects of allopathic drugs cause enormous problems, and as a result many patients are now seeking alternative approaches again (Astin 1998, Eisenberg 1993).

The increased use of alternative therapies has led to a call for more systematic data as evidence of effectiveness. This is difficult to provide because the elimination of complementary and alternative medicine from universities since around 1900 has meant that data have not been collected as systematically as they have been in 'orthodox' medicine (Coulter 1978). But mothers about to give birth to their children cannot wait until every treatment has passed scientific scrutiny in the form of a randomised clinical trial. The evidence of therapeutic results is a cornerstone of legitimacy for any therapy, but it is not always easy to acquire—particularly during pregnancy and labour. Not only are clinical trials expensive, but there are ethical difficulties about conducting trials, particularly drug trials, during pregnancy that stem from concerns for the well-being of the fetus. Moreover, the reality is that most medical interventions have not satisfied the rigours of a randomised control trial (Druss & Rosenheck 1999). On the other hand, patients want a basic certainty about effectiveness, cost and safety of any form of care they receive. How should this be provided if we do not have the evidence we would ideally like? What should be the source of evidence? Moreover, is practice legitimate only if it has fulfilled the demands of evidence-based medicine? Questioning the legitimacy of complementary medicine may be a sign of the general difficulty western society has in accepting other systems of thought as equally valuable; but at the same time science has not shown that complementary medicine is incommensurable with biomedicine (Astin 1998).

The historical developments confront us with another ethical aspect of midwifery: what is the legitimacy of practising within obstetrics a form of medicine with which many doctors are not familiar, but to which many midwives and women giving birth feel attracted? Gender issues also play a role here. Not long ago, the archetypal—male—obstetrician stood in a different relationship to the pregnant woman from the archetypal—female—midwife with less status (Fox Keller & Longino 1999). In the case of home births or in an outpatient setting in the hospital, the midwife and mother have acquired their respective autonomy. The midwife has the right to practise according to professional standards, and the woman has the right to decide on the setting of her delivery and the kind of treatments she prefers for herself and her baby.

These developments can create tensions for doctors who must accept both births in settings beyond their direct control and the unfamiliar complementary therapy techniques used there. In the UK, the Association of Radical Midwives (2002) has pointed to these parallel issues of autonomy.

Another issue concerns who is considered the expert on decisions about which form of medicine to apply—the professional or the patient. The traditional responsibility of doctors is seen in terms of beneficence, 'do no harm', and in a paternalistic model this can limit patients' autonomy if decisions are made unilaterally (Beauchamp & Childress 2001). Pregnancy and birth are particularly vulnerable in this respect as they are, in the western world, subjected to much medicalisation, making patient autonomy a scarce commodity.

Professional autonomy is limited by more than the simple fact of whether a technique is available or not. In the first place, a patient has to agree to its being used, but there is also a difference between whether a technique is available and whether the person considering using it has a thorough knowledge of the technique or training in its use. Likewise, availability is not the same as effectiveness, or even relative effectiveness. All these criteria must be met for good clinical practice to be possible. Education should be integrated, preferably into the current training programmes of midwives or additionally in postgraduate education. Research should be embedded in a holistic approach to evidence-based medicine. Why 'holistic'?

According to the principles of evidence-based medicine, evidence has its origin in two sources: systematic studies and the careful documentation of cases (Sackett 1996). In the case of homeopathy, the basis of its clinical practice is that the diagnostic and therapeutic principles of homeopathy are clearly described in textbooks; cases are documented in reports in journals; and systematic reviews are published (for instance Kleijnen et al 1991 and Linde et al 1997, as mentioned). In the following section, this body of knowledge is examined, together with the reasons for the controversy among doctors as to whether homeopathy is or is not 'scientific'—and this claim may form part of the legitimacy of practising medicine in the health care system of today.

This discussion will address the following in more detail: the principles of diagnosis and treatment of homeopathy, and its relationship with allopathic medicine; the research done in this domain; and the therapeutic responsibility that a midwife has in applying homeopathy within the context of professional competence.

FEATURES OF HOMEOPATHY

There are two basic features of homeopathy as a medical method that impact on allopathic or 'orthodox' medicine as traditionally taught in medical and paramedical education. These features are:

- at diagnostic level: the rule of similars and the individual diagnosis of a patient
- at therapeutic level: the use of high and ultra high dilutions ('dynamisations'). The process of dynamisation involves progressively diluting a substance in parts of 1 to 10 or 100 and shaking it vigorously with each step of dilution.

To date these features have been poorly understood (and explained) and have therefore led to controversies about homeopathy, which may be reduced if they are explained in contemporary scientific terms. They will be laid out in detail here, and in the next section their consequences in practice use will be illustrated.

The similarity rule

This rule states that a patient should receive a remedy made from a substance that can create in a healthy person the pattern of symptoms that is similar to the pattern of symptoms in the patient. This is often seen as strange, but it dates back to ancient Greek medicine.

In ancient Greece two medical traditions existed, the schools of Kos and Knidos. The first considered disease as an expression of disturbance of the 'dynamis', the self-healing power of any organism. Hippocrates, the founder of this tradition said: 'where there is a poison, there is a medicine' (Coulter 1975). He formulated the similarity rule that a medicine that can provoke illness in a healthy person should be given to a patient with a similar pattern of symptoms in order to cure them. Symptoms therefore have a guiding function; they reflect the specific actions of the defence mechanisms. This is the first form of a systemic approach to disease: the whole body participates in the effort to overcome the disease. The therapy is thus an 'imitation' of the disease. The reaction to this idea was embodied in the Knidos school whose followers tried to deduce all symptoms from one common cause, the 'disease entity'. According to this school, symptoms are alarm signs that need to be suppressed and therapy is an 'elimination' of the disease. This idea formed the basis of the western allopathic tradition, which in its search for this 'final cause', has yielded an enormous amount of knowledge on the pathological processes in our organs.

The beginning of homeopathy as a system of medicine can be traced to the innovations of Hahnemann, around 1800, when he began to conduct systematic experiments with healthy volunteers to register the 'pathogenetic effect' of many substances. By careful recording of these effects, a large number of substances, of animal, herbal and mineral origin, became available for medical treatment.

Medicines with minute doses

It is the use of minute doses in homeopathy that has sparked much of the controversy with allopathic medicine. Initially, for obvious ethical reasons, the substances were given only in minute doses to the healthy volunteers. Then it was discovered, purely empirically, that patients achieved a better cure if they received still lower doses. It seems that the historical conceptual differences played a much larger role than the discussion on high dilutions itself, as the debate started at a time when chemistry was still embryonic.

A general, material vision of nature such as developed in the 18th century apparently has inhibited a 'rapprochement', and Hahnemann's use of concepts such as 'vital force' did not make his ideas popular among his colleagues, who wanted to liberate medicine from non-material perspectives (Coulter 1978). But the recent advances in immunology and physics constitute a rational basis for understanding how low doses can work in a context of messengers circulating between organs. Histamine has been shown to exert a feedback on its own production in mast cells; and in dynamised preparation (shaken and diluted form), histamine still exerts this effect (Brown & Ennis 2001), which suggests that high dilutions have their effect through interaction with cellular receptors. Because activation of receptors does not depend on the quantity of a substance but on which substance contacts the receptor is confronted with, it does not depend on the amount but on the kind of substance.

Thus new scientific developments seem to provide data that can bridge the gap that developed in a time when our knowledge of the human organism was far more limited than now. So, how can these data be interpreted in a new model of disease?

Conceptual bridges

For reasons of safe patient care in obstetrics it is important to facilitate cooperation between professionals advocating different views. If some midwives already integrate homeopathy into their work and obstetricians in general do not, a conceptual model would be helpful to form a bridge between homeopathy and allopathy. Recent developments in immunology and endocrinology can link together a systemic and an organ perspective on disease: organs are ill because the information between them is disturbed (Eskinazi 1999). This information metaphor can create an opening for a new concept of disease: the 'biosemiotic model' where cytokines, hormones and neurotransmitters act as messengers connecting a network of interdependent organs (Brands et al 2000, Eder & Rembold 1992). With such a model in mind, practical cooperation in case management can take place, without the introduction of homeopathy being experienced as contradictory to current medical practice in obstetrics.

Selection of data for diagnosis

The main feature of homeopathic diagnosis and treatment on a practical level is the individual diagnosis: using patient features to find a remedy that 'fits the person' in order to treat the complaints of that person.

In general, two different strategies are used for attributing patients to disease categories:

- searching for the common features of a group of patients with the same main complaint and pathophysiological process, such as nausea in pregnancy or mastitis in the postpartum period. This is the strategy employed in allopathic medicine

- searching for the features by which patients with the same main complaint differ. They are then divided into subgroups; each group receives a diagnostic label, and as a consequence a different treatment. This is the strategy employed in homeopathy and Chinese medicine.

In homeopathy, a patient is compared with the 'remedy pictures' in the *Materia Medica*. These pictures have their origin in two sources. The first is the data from experiments (the experimental symptoms) and the second is the clinical symptoms because patients were treated with certain remedies if their pattern of symptoms was similar to the experimental one. Many clinical symptoms were added over the years. Together the two groups of symptoms form the prototype of a remedy: no person is identical to another who receives the same remedy, but they have enough similarity to be reckoned to be in 'the same family' (much as there are many different species of bird, but they form the collective family 'bird'). Psychology calls this 'family resemblance' (Rosch & Mervis 1975).

Diagnosis involves comparing one patient with a number of probable prototypes. This comparison is called 'differential diagnosis', and it is from this that the definitive choice is made. A similar process is used in all forms of medicine, with the choice of symptoms differing according to the principle under which they are organised: pathophysiology in allopathy, remedy picture in homeopathy and 'disease pattern' in Chinese medicine. The following division of data can help to distinguish between patients (Brands 1998).

A threefold registration of data

Type 1

The first group of data are those the patient has in common with others, for example stomach ache. Often those complaints are understandable from pathophysiology—that is, the process of deviant function of one or more specific organs. For instance, nightly stomach ache might occur in someone with a duodenal ulcer.

Type 2

There can also be complaints that are typical for a specific patient and that are not always understandable from pathophysiology. They are:

- typical sensations of the patient, e.g. a 'burning' stomach ache or the feeling 'as if a stone is lying on it'
- the concomitant or accompanying symptoms, such as headache or diarrhoea
- the 'modalities' or circumstances which aggravate or ameliorate the main complaint such as: time of the day, position of the body, pressure on the painful area, motion, etc
- aetiology: the circumstances that existed when the complaints started such as: fright, grief, nutritional changes, effects of cold or heat on the body.

Type 3

Finally there is a group of data that documents the typical features of the patient outside disease episodes. These are:

- mental features: impulsive, patient, expressive or repressive of emotions such as anger or grief
- general features: desire or aversion for certain food and drinks, reactions to humidity, cold, heat, motion, rest
- local features: symptoms that already existed at the onset of the main complaint, and previous diseases.

In both homeopathy and Chinese medicine this schema is used. The difference with allopathy is the use of patient-bound typical symptoms and features as obligatory elements in the choice of the disease category. Type 1 symptoms are often enough for the allopathic doctor but depend on additional data from laboratory investigations. Although homeopathy as a western form of medicine also uses pathophysiology as part of its conceptual model, it often has sufficient data for diagnosis with history and physical examination only. This is an advantage in situations that require rapid action when a laboratory is not available, and a home delivery is a good example of such a situation.

CASE MANAGEMENT OF SOME COMMON OBSTETRICAL PROBLEMS

Case management refers to the professional and responsible diagnosis, treatment and follow-up of a patient. It implies the correct choice of the indicated remedy, administering it, properly observing the reactions, and knowing what to do afterwards. It is reasonable to train midwives in homeopathic treatments as they already have highly developed skills of observation in pregnancy and delivery.

Midwives need to understand the following:

- which signs are to be noted
- indications and dosage
- eventual repetition of the remedy
- guidance, referral and collaboration.

What are the selection criteria?

A symptom is selected for diagnosis if it is intense and peculiar.

Intensity

Examples of intensity include the sensations of pain, fear, preferences for and aversions to certain types of food, and amelioration at certain points in the day. The subjective perception is important here, as in this respect patients have their own unique expertise. The signs perceptible to the professional can, however, complement these. The words of the woman must be registered precisely; for example, stomach ache described as a 'burning fire' is specific and informative as it indicates both the quantity and the quality of pain—it is not stitching or pressing.

Peculiarity

A symptom that is valuable for diagnosis must be 'peculiar'; that is, one that is remarkable, unusual or typical. This is because experiments and clinical experience have shown that peculiar symptoms are often good indicators for diagnosis. They convey information typical for the patient and it is this information, which distinguishes one person from another, that provides the distinction that leads to the correct choice of remedy.

Indications and dosage

Pregnancy and delivery are best regarded as naturally occurring processes, for which the midwife will not administer medicines too readily: 'respect for the physiology' is an important obstetrical attitude. This attitude applies equally to homeopathy. During the processes of pregnancy and birth, a woman has to be brought into equilibrium in order to proceed by her own potential (Geraghty 1997, Zaren 1989).

In order to justify an intervention with homeopathic medication, there must be clear signs of distress in either the mother or the fetus. They can be divided into the 'subjective' and the 'objective' aspects: the proper sensations of the woman and the externally observable features and symptoms.

The subjective condition of the mother

When looking at the subjective condition of the mother, a relatively easy cervical dilation phase and initially good contractions, for instance, leave the woman reasonably well off. Even if followed by a difficult labour, this history suggests less need for eventual intervention than if her reserves have already been used up during a difficult dilation and very painful and 'unproductive' contractions. There is still a long way to go, and the course of the labour is uncertain. Panic, pain and strong mood swings can be brought into balance by a remedy, and in this way the natural physiology of labour can be restored.

Objective criteria

The first objective criterion is the situation of the mother on examination or observation. Examples include alterations of position during pregnancy or delivery, and stagnating descent or non-effacement of the cervix during contractions. A problem with position can only exceptionally be influenced by homeopathy, which has been reported after the use of the remedy Pulsatilla but no further systematic studies have been done (Enkin et al 2002). Second, the situation of the child needs to be observed. Signs of fetal distress during delivery (meconium with decreasing heart rate) and the symptoms of the mother are signs both for the choice of remedy and for immediate referral to hospital. The rationale for administering the remedy is its rapid uptake through the circulation via the placenta, which may have a positive impact on the fetus.

Although the mother and child are considered to be one physiological entity, only the features of the mother can be observed—and during pregnancy features such as temperament, food desires or aversions or sleep patterns may change profoundly. If the mother does not show enough typical symptoms, remedies may be considered for a specific indication ('pathology prescribing'), for instance Carbo Vegetabilis (dynamised charcoal) for hypoxic situations.

The difference between the first and later phases of labour, the cervix dilatation and the expulsion, expresses itself in a different hierarchy between the two criteria—maternal distress and degree of infant deviation—which influence a decision about eventual intervention. During dilation, maternal distress is the first guiding criterion and infant deviation takes second place. During expulsion the order reverses; the deviation related to the child takes first priority and the maternal distress becomes the second priority.

For example, if a mother has a lot of pain (subjective sign) during a well-progressing dilation (objective sign), the attitude must be to wait before giving a remedy until the distress has reached an unacceptable degree. This differs, however, from when, during a painless expulsion (subjective sign), the head does not present sufficiently (objective sign). A rapid birth then becomes the first priority to prevent fetal distress. The situation of the fetus rather than that of the mother is the reason for the intervention.

How to start?

A starting point in homeopathy can be first to note down the typical symptoms on observation and questioning without giving a remedy, in order to establish the pattern recognition of a remedy. In the beginning it is wise to limit the use of remedies to those one knows well, and the indication for use should limit itself to acute situations at this stage, as typical symptoms (type 2) usually abound at this point. Chronic situations require more in-depth knowledge of those typical features (type 3 data) to select an appropriate therapy.

An example is the choice of remedies during difficult labour. They are grouped according to the level of excitation of the nervous system; this functions in a bipolar mode: excitation–inhibition. As this state can easily be observed, it is a major guideline to how to differentiate between remedies in this situation—some are indicated when the woman is very agitated, others when she is rather withdrawn.

Table 11.1 Remedies for difficult labour: central metaphors and main symptoms

Cimicifuga	Chamomilla	Belladonna	Ipecacuanha	Caulophyllum	Pulsatilla	Sabina	Secale	Kalic carbonicum	Sepia
Chaos	Overexcitation	Violent	Irritation	Rigidity	Changeable	Fear of loss	Weakness	Desire for control	Immobility
Coordination diminished	Touchy, angry, yelling	Delirium, anger, 'feverish'	Discontented	Changing moods	Gentle	Fear of losing the baby	Prostration, timidity	Strong sense of duty, attached to rules	Aversion to communication; sarcastic, joyless indifferent to loved ones
Talkative	'Purple from anger'	Head hot, extremities cold	Coughing in paroxysms with vomiting thereafter	Long and painful contractions without effect; closed cervix	Tearful alternating with laughing	Pain from sacral bone to pubic bone	Fears baby will die, suspicious of midwife	Fears felt in stomach	Rigidity of cervix
Rapid mood swings					Aversion to fats; desires cool drinks and open windows	Long profuse menstruation before pregnancy	Sensation: everything too loose, too open	Sensitive to draughts	Nausea from odours
Fear	Better by slow motion, or being borne, e.g. in a bath	Desire for cool drinks and cool applications							Chilly
Physical: spasms						Better lying on back	After birth: first remedy for haemorrhage	When touched contractions may stop	Better by exercise, strong movements

The main remedies are listed in Table 11.1. They range from very excited states—such as those corresponding to Cimicifuga—to depressed states such as in Sepia. These remedies have been used many times, so the reactions to them have been confirmed—some of them in randomised clinical trials (Kleijnen et al 1991, Linde et al 1997). The remedies listed here have partially provoked similar patterns in healthy people and have also cured symptoms in ill persons. Both groups of symptoms constitute their 'remedy pictures'. These pictures contain many symptoms from many organs. In order to understand in a basic way the effect a substance has on the organism, central metaphors are formulated to function as 'red threads' linking the different symptoms into a logical framework.

In Table 11.1, the central metaphors are mentioned first, then the main symptoms are listed. This is no more than a sample of the extended literature on these medicines, in order to facilitate a basic understanding of their different actions. This is the first step to making a differential diagnosis. Observation remains the start to practice.

References

Association of Radical Midwives 2002 Definition of normality. Online. Available: www.radmid.demon.co.uk

Astin J A 1998 Why patients use alternative medicine. Results of a national study. Journal of the American Medical Association 279:1548–1553

Beal M W 1998 Women's use of complementary and alternative therapies in reproductive health care. Journal of Nurse-Midwifery 43(3):224–234

Beauchamp T, Childress J 2001 Principles of biomedical ethics, 5th edn. Oxford University Press, Oxford

Brands M 1998 Disease, language and experience. A cognitive comparison of allopathy, homeopathy and Chinese medicine. Dissertation, Vrije Universiteit. Thela Thesis Publishers, Amsterdam

Brands M, Franck D, van Leeuwen E 2000 Epistemology and semiotics of medical systems: a comparative analysis. Semiotica 132(1/2):1–24

Brown V, Ennis M 2001 Flow-cytometric analysis of basophil activation: inhibition at conventional and homeopathic concentrations. Inflammation Research 50(supplement 2):S47–S48

Castro M 1992 Homeopathy for mother and baby. Macmillan, Basingstoke

Coulter H L 1975 Divided legacy. A history of the schism in medical thought, volume I. Wehawken Book Co, Washington DC

Coulter H L 1978 Divided legacy. A history of the schism in medical thought, volume III. Wehawken Book Co, Washington DC

Druss B G, Rosenheck R A 1999 Association between use of unconventional therapies and conventional medical services. Journal of the American Medical Association 282:651–656

Eder J, Rembold H 1992 Biosemiotics—a paradigm of biology. Naturwissenschaften 79:60–67

Eisenberg D M 1993 Unconventional medicine in the United States. North of England Journal of Medicine 328:246–252

Enkin M et al 2002 A guide to effective care in pregnancy and childbirth. Oxford University Press, Oxford

Eskinazi D 1999 Homeopathy re-revisited. Is homeopathy compatible with biomedical observations? Archives of Internal Medicine 159:1981–1987

Fox Keller E, Longino H 1999 Feminism and science. Oxford University Press, Oxford

Geraghty B 1997 Homeopathy for midwives. Churchill Livingstone, Edinburgh

Kleijnen J, Knipschild P, ter Riet G 1991 Clinical trials of homeopathy. British Medical Journal 302:316–323

Linde K et al 1997 Are the clinical effects of homeopathy placebo effects? A meta-analysis of placebo controlled trials Lancet 350:834–843

Prismant 1998 Continuous obstetrics registration. Illness Insurance Council (Ziekenfondsraad), Amsterdam

Prismant 2000 Continuous obstetrics registration. Illness Insurance Council (Ziekenfondsraad), Amsterdam

Rosch E, Mervis C 1975 Family resemblances: studies in the internal structure of categories. Cognitive Psychology 7:573–605

Sackett D 1996 Evidence based medicine: what it is and what it isn't. British Medical Journal 312:71–72

Zaren A 1989 Lelystad Seminar May 1989. Ilse Bos Publishers & Lutra Services, Amsterdam

PART 3

Professional issues

Chapter **12**

Midwifery autonomy and the code of professional conduct: an unethical combination?

Rachel Clarke[1]

The cruellest lies are often told in silence. (Robert Louis Stevenson)

INTRODUCTION

Deep in the psyche of midwifery lies the myth of the independent, autonomous practitioner. Belief in the myth is the result of a fractured reflection of midwifery's perception of itself that is rarely, if ever, questioned by midwives. Can midwives identify from whom or what they are independent? Can they demonstrate professional autonomy in an environment beset with policies, protocols and contractual obligations where their practice is as confined as the women they attend? The contrast between the myth of professional freedom and the observed control of midwives by the state, through employers and medicine, exposes the fallibility of the midwives' beliefs about their autonomous status in 20th-century childbearing.

---

[1] The chapter was updated by Heather Draper in March 2003 to take account of the new NMC Code of Conduct but the views expressed within the chapter are those of Rachel Clarke.

Despite the recommendations of *Changing Childbirth* (Department of Health 1993), the midwife is unlikely to achieve the status of an autonomous provider of maternity care without the aid of political and legal intervention. Present government policy is to leave the implementation of the recommendations to local NHS Trusts, rather than to intervene at a political or legislative level to overcome medicine's monopoly over maternity care.

This situation reflects the flaws in the Midwives Act 1902, which acknowledged the practitioner status of midwives, but failed to give them self-regulation (the right to define the scope of their professional authority and sphere of control). The rival profession of medicine was to have 'a dominant voice in their government' (Donnison 1988 p 174). Over the last 30 years the medicalisation of childbearing and the close association of midwifery with obstetrics have led to the obstetrician being acknowledged as the standard setter for midwifery practice. In the legal debate over the scope of practice it remains to be seen if traditional midwifery will be recognised by the courts as being superior to scientific biomedical obstetrics. Therefore, authentic professional autonomy has not been, and is unlikely to be, realistically within reach.

Until relatively recently midwifery autonomy was not an issue. Belief by midwives in its existence was harmless enough and it was of little consequence to obstetricians who continued to control childbearing events from conception to birth. However, two events served to highlight the tension between the real and imagined nature of professional autonomy for midwives. The first was the Nurses, Midwives and Health Visitors Act 1979, which established the United Kingdom Central Council (UKCC) as the statutory regulatory body for nurses, midwives and health visitors. The UKCC became fully functional in 1983, but was replaced by the Nursing and Midwifery Council (NMC) in 2002. The second event occurred in 1988 when a midwife in private practice, Jilly Rosser, was struck off the register by the UKCC for professional misconduct.

As part of its statutory duty to safeguard the public interest, and establish and improve standards of training and professional conduct for nursing and midwifery, the UKCC published the Code of Professional Conduct (UKCC 1992). This document introduced the professions to the concept of individual professional and moral accountability and the disciplinary framework that would be responsible for regulating professional conduct. An updated version of this document was produced by the NMC in 2002.

The Code is representative of a dimension of ethics known as prescriptive ethics, an approach which gives rise to policies, guidelines and codes of conduct/practice in an attempt to establish what one ought or ought not to do in practice. Such an approach further supposes that there is a definitive response to a situation and a definitive answer to a dilemma. In this respect the Code has not moved away from the historical legacy of strictly regulating the activities of nurses and midwives. In the past these professions have been overly concerned with attempting to standardise practice behaviour by using rules to prescribe right and wrong actions, rather than concentrating their efforts on identifying the dynamic nature of practice and the moral dimension of caring as a skilled, therapeutic activity. The Code of Professional Conduct exhibits what can only be called professional double-think, for it purports to be a document of principles, open to interpretation by informed, autonomous practitioners, when in truth it affirms the tradition of maintaining the homogeneous predictability of nursing/midwifery.

Underlying the assumption that practitioners are able to exercise professional and moral autonomy unfettered by the constraints of their employers and medical practitioners is a disregard for the true status of nurses and midwives as employees of the NHS. The professional mandate of the Code, arising from the statutory responsibility of the NMC, is to safeguard, promote and protect the interests of patients. This is a somewhat problematic mandate, given the restrictive nature of the role of nurses and midwives in the NHS.

In this chapter I argue that the NMC is profoundly unjust in expecting midwives to practise autonomously according to the requirements of the Code of Professional Conduct. Further, the Code is fundamentally flawed and therefore unethical for the following reason—it is based on the unwarranted assumption that midwives are autonomous practitioners professionally, clinically and morally.

Professional, clinical and moral autonomy are prerequisites for interpreting and following the Code's guidelines. Further, in order for midwives to be professionally accountable they must be professionally autonomous and it is on this basis that the NMC carries out its regulatory function of holding midwives accountable to the public in a fair and just manner. The fact that professional, clinical and moral accountability are not key features of midwifery practice, casts grave doubts upon the NMC's ability to perform this function.

OUTLINE OF THE CODE

The original UKCC Code was imposed on the workforce without consultation. Reg Pyne, the assistant registrar for standards and ethics at the UKCC when the Code was first published said that, 'there was no reason for the UKCC to be shy nor hesitant in its advice, nor did it have to dilute what is expected from practitioners or hold back from stating its view of the ideal' (Pyne 1987 p 30–31). He also suggested that the purpose of the Code was, 'to convert the profession from one that has seen good conduct as being compliant and submissive, to a profession that sees it as being more assertive and questioning' (Carlisle 1989 p 19). However, on the methods by which the professions of nursing and midwifery would be converted to these new values, the UKCC remained silent.

There was little evidence to support claims by the UKCC that the Code was a source of empowerment to practitioners and this led to widespread criticism of the Code. Tadd (1994) considered that the Code was simply an exercise in tokenism and wondered whether it had made any difference to the moral climate of nursing and midwifery.

The original Code used abstract concepts and ambiguous statements that were difficult to interpret, yet appeared deceptively simple to the unwary. For example, the first paragraph stated that each practitioner must, 'act always in such a manner as to promote and safeguard the interests and well-being of patients and clients'. The 2002 Code is more cautious, it only requires that practitioners 'protect and support the health of individuals patients and clients', though it goes on later to insist that the practitioner is 'personally accountable for ensuring that [he or she] promote and protect the interests and dignity of patients and clients' without discrimination. What does this really mean, and how far should a midwife go to safeguard these interests?

An example may help to illustrate the problem. A woman is about to undergo a planned, non-emergency caesarean section. Once under the anaesthetic, the obstetrician invites two or three junior doctors to perform vaginal examinations on her to add to their experience. The woman has not consented to these multiple examinations. When the midwife in theatre questions the ethics of this practice she is told by the obstetrician, 'What she doesn't know can't hurt her.' The midwife knows that examinations performed without consent constitute the civil tort of battery. She also knows that they are not in the woman's best interests, nor do they promote her dignity. What is she to do if she is to safeguard the woman's interests and dignity? This question has professional, moral and legal dimensions.

The Code of Professional Conduct states that each nurse, midwife and health visitor must:

- respect the patient or client as an individual
- obtain consent before any treatment is given

- protect confidential information
- cooperate with others in the team
- maintain professional knowledge and competence
- be trustworthy
- identify and minimise risk to patients and clients.

In trying to decide how the midwife might act in the foregoing example, difficulties in interpreting the Code become apparent. How is the midwife to promote the interests and dignity of the patient without exposing the unethical and illegal practice of the obstetrician? On the one hand she has obligations to her patient, and on the other she is required to cooperate with others in the team. However, the 2002 Code warns the practitioner that 'when working as a member of a team, you remain accountable for your professional conduct, any care you provide and any omission on your part' (section 4.5). Although also advised to act quickly to protect patients or clients from risk, this recommendation is made in the context of colleagues who may not 'be fit to practice for reasons of conduct, health or competence' (section 8.2), which is not obviously the case in this example, even though the intended conduct of the doctors is unethical and unlawful.

Due to its deceptive simplicity the moral nature of the Code has remained invisible to the majority of practitioners and so too have the dangers arising from simplistic interpretations, making the Code a dangerous document in the hands of the morally and politically naive. How is the interest or dignity of any patient to be defined and identified? What would happen if the midwife's interpretation of interest or risk clashed with the obstetrician's interpretation, as in the example given? Whose definition of interests or risk should be given precedence? The ramifications of these demands are enormous. Ideal practice, rather than good enough practice, is required by the Code, and the individual may be punished for failing to live up to this ideal, despite the constraints which make that ideal impossible to achieve.

When practitioners took issue with the then UKCC decision to strike them off the professional register and took their cases to court, the courts were critical of the UKCC and its idealistic expectations, in many instances ordering the UKCC to restore practitioners to the register. The attitude of the Courts was that the UKCC was too punitive in its enforcement of the idealistic standards of the Code of Professional Conduct (Flint 1989). It remains to be seen whether the same will be true of the NMC.

MIDWIFERY PRACTICE AND THE CONCEPT OF AUTONOMY

While there is little evidence to support the midwife's claim to professional autonomy, there is considerable evidence that it is undermined. Midwifery research has given us significant insights into the real nature of present-day practice that includes apathy, inertia and lack of control surrounding the exercising of clinical judgement and decision-making. These characteristics are a legacy of midwifery's modern development and it is here that we find the basis for midwifery dependency.

The impact of the Midwives Act 1902

The history of midwifery and women healers has been well chronicled. Achterberg (1991), Donnison (1988), and Garcia et al (1990) all capture the difficulties, the attitudes and the aspirations of the rival occupations of midwifery and obstetrics, charting the decline of midwifery and transformation of midwives into obstetric assistants during the 20th century.

The Midwives Act 1902 was a critical turning point for midwifery. It offered education, state registration and the prospect of respectability. It was welcomed with great warmth and enthusiasm by the Midwives Institute (first formed in 1880 as the Matron's Aid Society and now the Royal College of Midwives), whose primary aim was to raise the status of the occupation in order to attract middle-class women into the profession and improve standards, thereby offering greater protection to women in childbirth from incompetent midwives. There was, however, a price to be paid. In return for the continued tenure of midwifery, midwives not only had to accept a restricted sphere of practice that would be defined by medical men, they also had to surrender their professional autonomy.

The Central Midwives Board, created by the 1902 Act to regulate the education, training and registration of midwives, had no requirement to include midwives in its membership. Furthermore, when midwifery membership was finally granted in 1920, it was forbidden by statute for midwives to be in a majority. Medical practitioners had reason to be pleased; controlling midwifery education and practice through their influence on the Central Midwives Board would ensure that midwives stayed in their lowly and proper place. Not much had changed, it seemed from when it was said, 'what you want to educate midwives for is for them to know their own ignorance, that is really the one great object in educating midwives' (Select Committee on Midwives Registration, 1892, cited in Witz 1988 p 101).

Medical practitioners had drawn clear lines between what was midwives' work and what was doctors' work. The Midwives Institute accepted the division, making it quite clear they had every intention of working in harmony with doctors. Their betrayal of midwifery struck the most damaging blow to the achievement of full professional status. When the 1902 Act was passed, midwifery became a semi-profession and one subservient to medicine.

The 1902 Act preserved midwives in name, but reduced their competence and sphere of practice. They were left with the relatively unskilled role of attending at normal births, and the new rules made sure they called the doctor for any problem or face the possibility of losing their registration. Witz (1988) describes the method used to quell midwifery independence as a gendered strategy of de-skilling, demarcation and incorporation. It was spectacularly successful, for not only did midwives allow themselves to be manipulated into a position of subservience in 1902, they have never at any time later made any attempt to overthrow the oppressive influence of obstetrics. Obstetrics has continued to incorporate normal, healthy pregnant women into the medical domain and establish its credibility with the public by extolling the virtues of the scientific application of technology to achieve a safe birth.

The remainder of the 20th century saw a continued decline in midwifery skills and midwifery control in direct proportion to the growth of interventionist obstetrics and its philosophy that birth is only normal in retrospect. The effects of the decline in traditional midwifery skills and confidence have led to problems with the implementation of *Changing Childbirth* (DoH 1993), which appears to endorse freedom of choice by the consumer and a higher profile for midwives as the lead professional in the care of healthy childbearing women. Many midwives now feel unprepared and unwilling to accept this proposed level of responsibility (see Chapter 13).

Following the Nurses, Midwives and Health Visitors Act 1979, the UKCC took control of the education of nurses and midwives, restructuring it so that the medical influence was reduced. Nevertheless, in midwifery the medical obstetric influence endures through its emphasis on the pathology of childbearing and by the relentless, insidious destruction of traditional midwifery knowledge. Midwifery endorses this by default in approving obstetric units as suitable training establishments in which to learn midwifery. This legacy of subservience and powerlessness is responsible for the absence of professional, clinical and moral professional autonomy of midwives.

Professional autonomy and midwifery—some evidence

According to John Harris (1992) 'people are said to be autonomous to the extent to which they are able to control their own lives, and to some extent their own destiny, by the exercise of their own faculties' (p 195). Autonomy is not a commodity; it cannot be bought or sold or collected piecemeal. It is a characteristic of individuals who are able to direct their lives according to their own desires. For a professional group, autonomy is expressed in the way it defines and directs its own sphere of business/practice, provides appropriate education/training and monitors its members by a process of internal regulation without interference from others. Having endured control by the Central Midwives Board, which lacked adequate midwifery representation, midwifery now endures control by the NMC, which tends to include midwives under the generic term *nurses* and limits the influence of the Midwifery Committees set up to protect professional interests.

Significantly, the role of midwives continues to be defined by medical personnel and employers. Beauchamp & Childress (1994) state that autonomy must include 'personal rule of the self free from controlling interferences by others' (p 121). Nevertheless, controlling interferences continue to undermine midwives' opportunities to learn, achieve and exercise their full professional role. Harris cites four obstacles to autonomy, one of which is particularly useful when examining midwifery autonomy: 'defects in the individual's ability to control either her desires or her actions, or both' (Harris 1992 p 196).

The changes in midwives' role and responsibilities brought about by the increased medicalisation and hospitalisation of birth, further restricted the boundaries of their role, influenced the way they made decisions in the execution of their role and changed the way they perceived their role in relation to that of doctors. Influences on the education and training of midwives have altered the learning experience, so they have come to regard obstetric values and practices as representative of midwifery. As a result of these changes there are four areas of critical significance where there are serious defects in control: clinical practice, the clinical learning environment, ownership of the patient (accountability) and the exercise of clinical judgement. These will be considered in turn.

Clinical practice

The work of Robinson et al (1983) illustrated the lack of control that midwives have over their work. They observed that midwives frequently overestimated the extent to which they used their clinical judgement and seriously underestimated the extent to which obstetric policies exerted control over their decisions. This was particularly evident when caring for women in labour. Robinson et al are not alone in making these observations, Henderson (1984), Garcia et al (1985) and Garcia & Garforth (1991) have all demonstrated similar findings regarding some of the key areas of management of women in labour; for example, performing vaginal examinations; deciding to rupture the membranes; and deciding to use electronic fetal monitoring.

The traditional practice of performing 4-hourly vaginal examinations is a particularly interesting one, for no work has been done to support the value of such a regime. Its purpose is to produce conformity to the obstetric partogram (a graph on which all labour events are charted), in order to give an illustrated progress report on labour. In performing this 4-hourly procedure, which is unnecessary, invasive and unevaluated, midwives reveal a marked lack of professional and clinical autonomy. It is extremely doubtful that midwives would now be willing to forgo the routine 4-hourly vaginal examination in favour of skilled abdominal assessment, due to the lack of skill and confidence induced by exposure to obstetric influence and the general fear of litigation.

One of the disturbing features of Robinson's study (Robinson et al 1983) was the degree of acquiescence that midwives demonstrated to doctors taking over completely, or replicating the most basic aspects of their role. The data showed a substantial number of midwives never had an opportunity to rely entirely on their own skills and judgements in assessing the course of pregnancy, because the medical staff took over this responsibility. Yet this is an aspect of practice which is fundamental not only to the role of midwives, but to their very existence. In the key area of abdominal examination, almost all midwives in the study felt that this was a task appropriate for the midwife, yet almost all the hospital midwives and two- thirds of community midwives worked in situations where the doctor carried out this examination and, despite this, an astonishing

60% of hospital midwives and 72% of community midwives felt this division of responsibility was about right (Robinson et al 1983).

Despite the reassuring confirmation that the midwife is the person who delivers over 70% of babies, it is optimistic to take this statistic as an indicator of professional autonomy. Even here, management of key areas such as the length of the second stage of labour and the method of delivery of the placenta and membranes are controlled by arbitrary obstetrically derived time limits and methodology (see Chapter 5). Evidence of the erosion of midwifery skills arising from the medicalisation of labour became evident in the Bristol Third Stage Trial, a research study that set out to compare outcomes of different management approaches to the third stage of labour (Inch 1990). The declaration that the trial was invalid was due, in part, to the lack of knowledge and skill of the midwives who were assigned to conduct normal, physiological delivery of placenta and membranes. In short, they did not know how. Their training as students and their practice as qualified midwives had never enabled them to gain expertise in traditional midwifery skills, one of which is the management of a completely physiological delivery of placenta and membranes.

Since Robinson et al's (1983) work there has been no similar study to re-assess the midwife's role in the UK, but there is little reason to suppose any fundamental change has occurred. Following the publication of *Changing Childbirth* (DoH 1993), the Royal College of Obstetricians and Gynaecologists made it clear that its members were opposed to the proposed changes, which include making the midwife the lead professional in the care of normal, healthy women. They wanted the term 'lead professional' replaced by 'link professional'. They questioned the reduced input from obstetricians in the care of normal women (which they said was unacceptable) and they expressed the fear (perhaps tongue-in-cheek) that midwives may become isolated if they become independent practitioners (Dunlop 1993). The root of this conflict lies in delineating professional power, and the midwife's role will not change significantly while obstetricians continue to exert control over childbearing events.

The effects of the learning environment

Training schools for midwives must be approved by the appropriate National Board (part of the statutory structures set up by the 1979 Act to assist the UKCC). It is not just the educational establishment that must be approved; the obstetric unit in which students gain their practical experience must also be approved.

The irony is that midwives have such a lack of control over their own education that they give approval to obstetric units as suitable places to learn normal, traditional midwifery skills. These are the very places where such experience is either unavailable or so infrequently available that no student or midwife could accumulate sufficient experience to claim to be an expert in normal (physiological) childbearing events. In obstetric units students of midwifery find it impossible to witness 10 deliveries of women whose labours were completely physiological, followed by their supervised personal management of 40 further cases, also completely physiologically normal. It is not surprising that the work of Robinson et al (1983) and the results of the Bristol trial demonstrated such a marked and fundamental shift in the knowledge and skills of midwives. If midwifery approves the placing of students in obstetric units where what they learn is obstetrically oriented, it must accept responsibility for the outcome—that is, midwives who are ill-prepared and reluctant to accept the validity of midwife-led, low-technology, low intervention care outside the confines of a medically oriented unit. The lack of control in this key area of midwifery is crucial to understanding why midwives are generally unwilling and unable to take control of the management of childbearing women.

Ownership of the patient and accountability

There is a third, equally critical area, where midwives exhibit lack of control. Like the old Code, the 2002 Code repeatedly requires the practitioner to protect, promote and support the interests of individual patients and clients. Safeguarding these interests, which are left to the practitioner to define, frequently brings the individual into conflict with medical staff and employers. Graham Pink famously attempted to follow the old UKCC Code to draw attention to gross understaffing which, he claimed, resulted in poor patient care. His case graphically illustrated to nurses and midwives their isolated and helpless status. While the investigating committee of the English National Board for Nursing, Midwifery and Health Visiting decided not to refer Pink's case to the UKCC, his employers found him guilty of gross professional misconduct, a situation in which the UKCC was unable to intervene effectively (Carlisle & Hempel 1991).

Whistleblowing, especially by nursing staff, has never been popular in the NHS but this is exactly what practitioners are required to do in their patients' best interests, regardless of the consequences for the individual practitioners concerned.

Consider the following case based on real events. A consultant obstetrician, who is fervently anti-abortion, nevertheless offers amniocentesis to a woman. During the procedure, he deliberately draws off an insufficient amount of amniotic fluid to enable the laboratory staff to perform the tests that will determine possible abnormality of the fetus. The midwife knows what he has done and she has seen him do this on every other occasion she has assisted him at the procedure. By the time the woman returns for her results it is too late for a repeat test. The midwife knows that it is a ploy on his part to avoid the possibility of termination if the test indicates there is fetal abnormality.

The Code requires this midwife to act in a way that safeguards and protects the patient's interests. There are two issues here: first, the midwife does not have a patient, the patient *belongs* to the consultant who alone has the legitimate authority to diagnose, treat and discharge the patients. How can she act in the patient's best interests when, in effect, she has no patient and no authority to act on her behalf? Second, the UKCC, and subsequently the NMC, have burdened practitioners with the *moral* ownership of patients and demands that they carry moral responsibility for them. If the midwife in this example tells the woman what has happened she might choose to go elsewhere for her antenatal care and she might also complain loudly about the reason why. In the past, the midwife would almost certainly have put herself at risk of being charged with gross professional misconduct by her employer and even of dismissal for lowering the integrity of the medical staff in the eyes of the patient by disclosing this information. The introduction of the Public Interest Disclosure Act 1998, might go some way to alleviating this problem, but there are no guarantees that this will be the case. It is interesting that while the NMC web site (accessed 18 March 2002) contained publications explaining how to complain about NMC registered practitioners, it offered no similar guidance to members about legitimate whistleblowing or how to do this legally.

There are other examples that exemplify the power differential between medical staff and midwives. When a woman is pregnant with twins and one of them has a condition that is incompatible with life, it is the doctor alone who has the power to decide if the woman is to be told. The midwife must continue to provide midwifery care within this wall of silence. Authentic midwifery has become invisible within obstetrics and midwives are permitted only to provide midwifery care as it is defined by obstetrics; that is, carry out those routine observations and monitoring tasks that do not require, and indeed prevent, the establishment of professional intimacy and responsibility. Even if midwives in such a case believe they have a moral duty to inform the woman of the situation, they dare not do so; the doctor's decision is final and the midwife does not have the authority to overturn the clinical judgement of the doctor (Dimond 1990).

Evidence of defects in control continue to be a feature of the institution of midwifery and of midwifery practice and seriously undermines the claim that midwives are professionally autonomous. The evidence also casts doubt on the assumption of the NMC that midwives have the professional, clinical and moral autonomy necessary to practise as directed by the Code of Professional Conduct.

Clinical judgement and the case of Jilly Rosser

The case of Jilly Rosser who, in 1988, was found guilty of gross professional misconduct and struck off the register by the UKCC, illustrated the idealistic nature of the Code of Conduct and the attitude of the UKCC to the professional autonomy of midwives.

The evidence of misconduct against Rosser included criticism of her record keeping and her decision to transfer a patient (who was haemorrhaging, following a birth at home) to hospital in her own car rather than wait for the emergency services to arrive. In response to the charge about her records, Rosser claimed that they were made as the situation permitted, in accord with Rule 42 of the *Midwives Rules*, which among other things states that records will be made, 'as contemporaneously as is reasonable' (UKCC 1993 p 21). In response to the second charge regarding the use of her own car to transport the patient to hospital, Rosser claimed that her professional knowledge and experience of the poor performance of the emergency services in responding to calls enabled her to predict with a high degree of certainty that her patient's condition would deteriorate significantly if she waited for them to arrive. With this local knowledge and her midwifery experience, Rosser arrived at a clinical decision that she believed best served her patient's interests.

Rosser's clinical decision was not accepted by the Professional Conduct Committee of the UKCC, who declared her guilty of professional misconduct and removed her name from the register. Rosser was unhappy with this judgement and took the case to the High Court. It was hoped that the judge, Lord Justice Watkins, would interpret the meaning of misconduct but his judgement was not heard because the UKCC, in what Flint (1989) called a 'face-saving exercise', conceded the case and withdrew. Rosser was allowed her appeal and the UKCC was ordered to reinstate her on the register.

During the case, Lord Justice Watkins questioned the unrealistic expectations of the UKCC regarding midwives' capabilities. It was his opinion that Rosser's records were satisfactory up until the time of the emergency but, he pointed out, she would then have been engaged in examining her patient, contacting the patient's general practitioner and arranging for her transfer to hospital. The barrister acting for the UKCC claimed that Rosser should have been jotting down notes while holding the patient's hand, to which Lord Justice Watkins replied, 'she would have to be a first class juggler'. Lord Justice Watkins went on to say that he found the charge against Rosser resulting from her decision to take the patient to hospital in her own car to be perverse, and asked the UKCC's barrister if Rosser would be in the same situation if she had passively waited for the emergency services to arrive. Clearly, Watkins suspected that she could then have been charged with professional misconduct for failing to safeguard the patient's best interests by taking her to hospital in her own car.

In the absence of any statement from the UKCC clarifying the exact nature of Rosser's misconduct, one might be forgiven for supposing that the motives of the UKCC might have been more to do with curtailing midwifery independence than protecting the public. Significantly, the law did not find any aspect of Rosser's practice unusual or unsafe. Rosser had to make a decision about what action on her part might best safeguard and promote her patient's best interests in accordance with the Code of Professional Conduct. Specifically, she had to decide whether, given the performance of the local emergency services, it was in her patient's best interests to wait and bleed, perhaps to death, or to be transported to hospital by any means available and as quickly as possible in order to safeguard her life. Her decision seems to reflect the assertiveness and questioning that Reg Pyne (1987) claimed the Code sought to promote.

Clinical judgement is just that, a judgement; it is not a definitive rule that can be written down as an action plan for others to follow. It varies according to the situation and people involved and the practitioners' responses to them, and the way in which the Code is written seems to reflect this. But if the UKCC wanted practitioners to interpret and act on those principles, why did it punish Jilly Rosser for doing exactly that? It is hardly surprising that many practitioners believe the Code could be used to damn them whatever they do.

MAINTAINING MIDWIVES' LACK OF AUTONOMY

Let us suppose that midwives were to be granted the same authority as doctors to make clinical decisions without the constraints of protocols and procedures and to act with complete professional autonomy. Given the current structure of care it is not difficult to imagine circumstances where the result would be a clash between two professionally autonomous practitioners, each with a different view about the clinical management of a particular pregnant woman. One way of resolving this problem is to ensure that one profession or the other is given less authority. Arguably it is not in the public interest for patients to be fought over, or to become pawns in an interprofessional battle for control. What has yet to be established, however, is why it is midwives who should have the lesser authority or why some other mechanism—perhaps more genuine team working—could not be established to resolve the potential problem.

CONCLUSION

A regulatory authority like the NMC must be able to justify how its Code of Conduct can be implemented in practice. The NMC should justify how its members can both adhere to the Code and be employees in an environment that curtails autonomous professional decision-making. The NMC has little influence over the contractual environment in which its members practice. It is unreasonable for professional registration to be contingent on following a Code of Practice that can potentially damn one whatever one decides to do. It is unacceptable for midwives to feel that it is better to ignore patients' best interests in order to safeguard their own, but it is equally unacceptable for midwives to have to risk becoming martyrs to protect their patients' interests and dignity.

References

Achterberg J 1991 Woman as healer. Rider, London
Beauchamp T L, Childress J F 1994 Principles of biomedical ethics, 4th edn. Oxford University Press, Oxford
Carlisle D 1989 Silence is not golden. Nursing Times 85(36):19
Carlisle D, Hempel S 1991 Conduct unbecoming? Nursing Times 87(30):18
Department of Health Expert Maternity Group 1993 Changing childbirth (the Cumberledge Report). HMSO, London
Dimond B 1990 Legal aspects of nursing. Prentice Hall, London

Donnison J 1988 Midwives & medical men. Historical Publications, London

Dunlop W 1993 Changing childbirth—commentary II. British Journal of Obstetrics and Gynaecology 100:1072–1073

Flint C 1989 A matter of judgement. Nursing Times 85(12):19

Garcia J, Garforth S 1991 Midwifery policies and policymaking. In: Robinson S, Thomson A (eds) Midwives, research & childbirth volume II. Chapman & Hall, London

Garcia J, Garforth S, Ayers S 1985 Midwives confined? Labour ward policies and routines. In: Research & the midwife conference proceedings 1985. Nursing Education Research Unit, Kings College, London

Garcia J, Kilpatrick R, Richards R 1990 The politics of maternity care. Clarendon Paperbacks, Oxford

Harris J 1992 The value of life: an introduction to medical ethics. Routledge, London

Henderson C 1984 Influences and interactions surrounding the midwife's decision to rupture the membranes. In: Research & the midwife conference proceedings 1984. Nursing Education Research Unit, Kings College, London

Inch S 1990 The Bristol third stage trial. Association for the Improvement of Maternity Services (AIMS) Quarterly Journal 1:8–10

Nursing and Midwifery Council 2002 Code of conduct. Online. Available: www.nmc-uk.org

Pyne R 1987 A professional duty to shout. Nursing Times 83(42):30–31

Robinson S, Golden J, Bradley S 1983 A study of the role and responsibilities of the midwife. Nursing Education Research Unit, Kings College, London

Tadd V 1994 Professional codes: an exercise in tokenism? Nursing Ethics 1:15–23

United Kingdom Central Council (UKCC) 1992 Code of professional conduct. UKCC, London

United Kingdom Central Council (UKCC) 1993 Midwives rules. UKCC, London

Witz A 1988 Patriarchal relations and patterns of sex segregation. In: Walby S (ed) Gender segregation at work. Open University Press, Milton Keynes

Chapter **13**

Retention and autonomy in midwifery practice

Alison Ledward

INTRODUCTION

The recommendations of *Changing Childbirth* are based on the principle of autonomy. A major focus of the report was the promotion of 'woman-centred' care (Department of Health 1993 p 5). A further distinctive element was the expansion of the midwife's professional autonomy (Department of Health 1993 p 39). Against this background, this chapter aims to examine some of the ethical issues raised in the light of the current retention crisis in midwifery. It will be argued that there are conflicts in practice between the recommendations of *Changing Childbirth* and the experience of midwives. The reasons for this are, I think, twofold. First, *Changing Childbirth* did not address the fact that midwifery practice is frequently constrained by policies and protocols that are obstetrically driven. Second, the new, more innovative types of care might result in some instances in midwives having to forfeit a degree of autonomy. It will be argued that these factors have exacerbated the retention crisis in midwifery. This has important consequences for the way in which women are treated. Fewer practising midwives may result in less care for women and may increase the use of medical intervention and technology on women whose clinical condition does not warrant it.

AUTONOMY

Beauchamp and Childress define autonomy as 'self-rule' and freedom from the influences of others (1994 p 120–121). Autonomy is valuable as it enables individuals to set and achieve their own goals. However, valuable as autonomy is, there are other ethical principles and it should not always be assumed that autonomy is the most valuable principle of all. No one is fully autonomous but, as we shall see, there are varying degrees of autonomy.

AUTONOMY IN RELATION TO MIDWIFERY PRACTICE

Symon (1996) argues that 'any reasonable concept of an autonomous group would preclude that group having its standards of practice determined to any great extent by another group' (p 547). Midwifery practice could not claim to be unaffected by interference by obstetricians and managers and this interference may unnecessarily restrict midwives' clinical freedom. For example, there are pressures to conform to protocols and to view pregnancy and birth as abnormal. Organisational factors, which are often devised with the smooth running of the establishment in mind rather than the best interests of the women, may further undermine midwives' professional autonomy.

Opportunities for midwives

Midwives were, in theory, invited by *Changing Childbirth* to seize the opportunity to expand their professional role and assume responsibility as the lead professional in the care of women whose pregnancies were normal, for such is their professional domain. It should be stressed that midwife-led care includes a socially supportive element in addition to the physical aspects of a woman's care.

On the face of things, the time was ripe for midwives to exercise a high degree of professional autonomy. Never at any time in the past had midwives had conferred on them such long-awaited opportunities to expand their professional role. Under-utilisation of the midwife's skills was to become something relegated to the past.

The midwife's role would mirror the assertion of the UKCC *Midwives rules and code of practice* that '[a] practising midwife is responsible for providing midwifery care to a mother and baby during the antenatal, intranatal and postnatal periods' (1998 p 17). *Changing Childbirth* emphasised that pregnant women should also have more control over their maternity care. The fact that it was considered to be in the interests of pregnant women for the role of midwives to change, added further ethical impetus. Theoretically, therefore, both pregnant women and midwives stood to benefit from the changes through increased autonomy.

LIMITS ON MIDWIVES' PROFESSIONAL AUTONOMY

Midwives' professional autonomy is not, however, limitless and nor should it be. They have to work with other professionals and recognise the limits of their own professional competence. For instance, in the case of a breech presentation, it may be in the best interests of the woman to hand over her care to an obstetrician. The limits of professional competence and autonomy are easier to agree in principle than practice as sometimes midwives and obstetricians may disagree about a particular management decision or policy even though both parties recognise the expertise and skills of the other. The professional autonomy (and role) of midwives is, however, undermined when obstetrics intrudes into the care of uncomplicated, low risk, normal pregnancies.

Changing Childbirth did not address the pre-existing constraints placed on midwives' autonomy by hospital policies and protocols. Although such policies and protocols are designed to protect women and health care professionals, they are frequently obstetrically driven and not necessarily evidence-based. The drive to promote the autonomy of women and midwives through the implementation of a new schema of care which, although organisationally diverse, shares a 'woman-centred' philosophy, is consistent with midwives' professional code of conduct. Paragraph 7 of the *Code of Professional Conduct* specifies that the midwife should provide care that is woman focused (UKCC 1992). The midwife's employer, however, may stipulate that care be provided in line with the particular NHS Trust's protocols. If midwives disagree with their Trust's protocols in a particular case, they face a dilemma. They can make the woman in their care a 'special case', in which the protocols do not apply, and by so doing they retain their professional autonomy. Alternatively, they can conform to their Trust's protocol, thereby forfeiting some of their professional autonomy and also depriving the patient of her chosen option.

This dilemma is best illustrated with reference to a case in practice. Consider the following. A midwife is caring for a woman whose labour is normal. It has been agreed that the woman wishes to avoid artificial rupture of the membranes (ARM), unless clinically indicated, as she perceived it as very painful last time. The midwife defines the presenting part as 'high cavity' on vaginal examination, in which case ARM would not be in the best interests of either the woman or her fetus. Accordingly, the woman and midwife await spontaneous rupture of the membranes (SRM). However, it is the local NHS Trust's policy to perform ARM at 4 cm dilatation of the cervix because intact membranes may delay the progress of labour. The midwife ignores the policy, choosing instead to follow her professional judgement that ARM is inappropriate. In so doing, she is also promoting what the woman herself wants but she may place herself at risk of being disciplined by her employer for not following the established protocol. Not surprisingly, some midwives feel that while they are professionally accountable for the care they give, they do not have the authority to act on their professional judgements.

It has been acknowledged that health care professionals are beset by constraints that influence working practices. *Making a Difference* noted that professionals are 'often constrained by structures that limit development and innovation' (Department of Health 1999 p 13). However, the report goes on to recommend that 'there is scope for midwives to apply their knowledge and skills more widely' (Department of Health 1999 p 66). Whether or not newly acquired professional responsibilities represent increased autonomy for midwives is open to debate. Bradshaw & Bradshaw (1997) commenting on the views of Harrison & Pollitt (1994) warn against midwives assuming that taking responsibility for tasks (like intravenous cannulation) that were previously the responsibility of junior doctors is 'a sign of upward occupational mobility'. Rather, they claim, this demonstrates medicine's dominance over midwifery: it is the *obstetrician* who thereby defines the parameters of the midwife's role. This is because it is assumed that as medical knowledge is superior to midwifery knowledge, so that the application of midwifery skills must be authorised by an obstetrician.

An alternative view might be that in accepting the extension to their role, midwives are acting more autonomously, but this is suspect since midwifery is a defined sphere—midwives are not quasi-obstetricians. Recognising the different roles does not, however, mean that seeking advice from an obstetrician limits a midwife's autonomy; rather each professional brings a different type of expertise to bear in order to benefit the woman.

In this climate, it would seem crucial that newly acquired skills should promote 'normality' in midwifery practice. Equally, the apparent increase in career opportunities should be viewed with caution. Positions offering midwives 'specialist' practitioner status may be the response of medicine and management to the retention crisis in midwifery. Exercising control over midwives' autonomy in the guise of seemingly attractive career packages that are superficially 'enabling' to the midwives' professional role may be at best tokenistic and at worst, illusory. Mounting pressures on heads of midwifery to recruit and retain midwives has resulted in the creation of posts in some centres that denote seniority and leadership within the profession. Strong leadership is commendable, but some midwives might feel that making midwifery more hierarchical places their professional autonomy under further threat. The cultural environment of midwifery remains predominantly unchanged and those midwives engaged in the new roles may find themselves subject to the same constraints as other midwives. However, in the long-term, it is possible that the implementation of such posts could help to promote equity between midwives and obstetricians.

THE CURRENT RETENTION CRISIS IN MIDWIFERY

There can be little doubt about the retention crisis in midwifery. According to O'Dowd (2000) as many as 60 000 registered midwives are out of practice. Furthermore, there is recent evidence that the situation is deteriorating. The Royal College of Midwives (2002) claims that

> More units than ever before, including more than 9 out of 10 units in England, are currently carrying unfilled posts. The overall and long-term vacancy rates are the highest we have ever recorded. Furthermore, vacancy rates have increased across every county and region other than London where it remains at a critically high level—and Northern Ireland. (p 17)

The situation persists despite a national drive to increase the number of practising midwives.

The link with autonomy

According to Stafford (2001) '[t]here is possibly a link between lack of autonomy and midwives leaving the profession' (p 46). This she attributes to many midwives being unclear about the extent of their own sphere of practice and their inability to provide training programmes and self-regulation intraprofessionally. Some midwives feel frustrated by the theory/practice gap, feeling forced to practise according to obstetrically driven protocols that are not necessarily evidence-based. She may have a valid point. Some midwives, sincere in their quest to practise woman-centred care and promote the interests of women, may feel frustrated by what they perceive as unwarranted constraints on their clinical freedom. Arguably, if *Changing Childbirth* was seen as a breakthrough from the traditional, medically dominated types of care, then it should follow that 10 years later, midwives should have had time and opportunity to become more autonomous in their professional domain. Although *Changing Childbirth* offered an impetus for change that should benefit women and midwives, the emerging picture is that, far from being able to plan care that is appropriate for women, midwives cannot utilise the services to meet women's preferences and concerns. The infrastructure needed to support midwives' autonomous practice is absent. Midwives are essentially caught in the crossfire. The retention crisis may only serve to highlight the dichotomy between the recommendations of *Changing Childbirth* and life at the coalface for midwives. Crucially, midwives should be involved in the planning, implementation and evaluation of women's care. It is they who should be assessing the effectiveness of midwifery interventions and using their assessments as a basis for evidence-based midwifery intervention in lieu of obstetric protocol, where appropriate. It is initiatives such as these that will enhance midwives' professional autonomy.

Midwives' autonomy frustrated rather than promoted

There may be grounds for saying that some midwives' autonomy has been subjected to restrictions. As Kirkham (1999) puts it '[m]idwives who are expected to facilitate choice and control for clients often lack professional experience of such facilitation, exercise little choice and control in their work and mistrust management' (p 737). Midwifery care should promote childbearing as a natural event and combine that philosophy with options that meet women's rather than obstetricians' preferences. Working within this framework, midwives should be able to balance the appropriate use of technology against non-intervention. Midwife-led care should enable the woman to extend her horizons beyond the medical confines of pregnancy and to decide which elements of care are important to her.

The reality of the situation is that midwives are trained in an obstetrically oriented environment. It is therefore not surprising that midwifery care for the normal pregnant woman is frequently enmeshed with the type of care designed for women whose clinical condition is complicated. Working within these parameters, it is difficult for midwives to extend their autonomy. This is amply demonstrated by Shallow (2001) who maintains that midwives' competencies in the care of normal pregnant women are compromised by undue pressure being exerted to view all births as abnormal. She concludes that '[m]any midwives have become so socialized in hospital methods of working that they have all but lost sight of what is fundamental to midwifery practice'(p 243). Shallow's view is consistent with the fact that some midwives endeavoured to implement the recommendations of *Changing Childbirth* but were thwarted by influences from the medical establishment (Harcombe 1999). This may originate from a culture in which doctors were seen as the experts, with the result that their powers were subsequently enhanced (Barbour 2001). In addition, there were different perceptions of the new care types; they were viewed by some as elitist because they considered that those engaged in them theoretically enjoyed higher levels of autonomy. The rhetoric of the situation, as we shall see, is that some midwives were obliged to forfeit some degree of their autonomy in clinical areas outside their designated area of midwifery practice.

Providing the type of care the woman wants within reasonable ethical boundaries represents a challenge for midwives. Some midwives would positively rise to the challenge but even if the outcome for the woman and her baby is good in the physical sense, midwives may still have negative feelings about the experience if, for example, they were restricted by a protocol that is difficult to support. Sometimes research-based evidence may refute current practice, for instance continuous monitoring of the fetal heart rate throughout normal labour (Walsh 2000). The decision to implement an intervention such as this should be reached as a process of negotiation between the woman and the midwife on an individual case-by-case basis, and the absence of this negotiation can lead some midwives to feel uncertain about whether or not to implement monitoring. However any attempt to change traditional practices can seem quite radical and requires commitment from both midwives and managers. The general situation may be aggravated further by a lack of consensus among midwives about the effectiveness of an intervention and because obstetricians sometimes vigorously defend their professional role. Midwives who fail to receive the necessary support to implement evidence-based changes to their working practices may feel that their professional autonomy is frustrated, and some midwives may view the situation as being inequitable. Sometimes managers are seen as integral to the problem. Midwives, disillusioned when their judgements are disputed or even refuted out of hand without justification, may elect to leave the profession for these reasons. Effective communication between midwives and managers can be a way of avoiding conflict. In order to motivate and sustain midwives, it would seem crucial that a forum is created in which boundaries are respected and midwives feel more able to influence their work environment and practices relating to the care of the normal pregnant woman. As Stafford (2001) points out, midwife involvement in decision-making and planning and the opportunity to provide the care for which they were trained, given the current retention crisis, would be a wise investment (p 47).

MIDWIVES' EXPERIENCES

A major study entitled *Why Do Midwives Leave* (Ball et al 2002) draws on the research undertaken by the University of Sheffield's Women's Informed Childbearing and Health Research Group. Their research was based on 28 in-depth interviews and a questionnaire completed by 978 midwives who ceased to practice in 1999/2000. It should be emphasised that the various reasons midwives leave the profession are complex, but there is strong evidence from the study that 'dissatisfaction with midwifery' (p 38) was the major factor for many deciding to leave.

The predominant feature of the research was the strong sense of diminished professional autonomy felt by midwives working with the new care types both in the hospital and the community. As one midwife respondent put it:

> I said you're wanting midwives to be jack of all trades ... you can't have a midwife who can do all that. The omnipotent midwife ... I think you're asking too much of her. G. Grade Midwife. (Ball et al 2002 p 17)

I have already argued that midwives have never had full professional autonomy. It would be difficult to dispute, however, that some midwives may be more autonomous in certain areas of clinical practice than in others. The resultant effect means that midwives may surrender a degree of professional autonomy in one area of practice in order to increase it in another less familiar area. For example, a midwife whose main clinical competencies are in antenatal care may be obliged to rotate to the postnatal ward where being less familiar with the work patterns means the midwife is unable to demonstrate the same level of competency as in the antenatal area of work. The English National Board (1995) concedes that a midwife cannot be an expert in every area, but each midwife should be professionally and legally '[at least] reasonably competent' (p 9). It is, though, difficult to see how midwives can attain this reasonable level of competence when current practice obliges them to rotate between all areas of midwifery practice. Moreover, any newly acquired level of competence, for example perineal suturing, needs to be sustained through practice. Hence, the mechanisms of the organisation of care have the potential to enhance or restrict a midwife's professional autonomy by the way in which they either promote or restrict the acquisition of skills. Midwives themselves are also guilty of eroding the professional confidence, and therefore autonomy, of their colleagues. For example, a community midwife's skills in the provision of home birth to women in her locality may be derided during her rotation in the hospital by a labour ward midwife regularly working on the fringe of technology. In this type of situation, not only is the community midwife's autonomy restricted in the labour ward, but her notions of what counts as a reasonable level of autonomy in the community may also be crushed, affecting her practice on her return to the community.

Changing Childbirth recommended that the midwife is 'able to work across a variety of settings' (Department of Health 1993 p 38). However, respect for the limitations on midwives' autonomy, which may paradoxically occur, are given only cursory attention. If midwives' decision-making skills are affected by working in this way, it follows that it may place restrictions on their potential for greater professional autonomy. From this account, we may deduce that the new types of care that may include enforced rotation contribute to midwives' decision to leave. As Ball et al say '[m]idwives who were significantly more likely to feel they did *not* have enough control over how their work was organised were those who worked in hospital/community integrated teams. 61% worked in a combination of *all* clinical areas' (Ball et al 2002 p 53). What is significant is that midwives practising in this way felt disempowered by the restrictions placed on their autonomy and this influenced their decision to leave. Enforced rotation certainly seems to be contributing to midwives leaving the profession.

Different constraints

Some centres, however, elected to retain 'core' midwives in clinical areas, which means they are permanent and not rotated. These midwives should retain their previously acquired professional autonomy in their designated area of practice. This is arguably unfair on other midwives who, by nature of their contractual obligations, must rotate on a regular basis. On the other hand, even in a clinical environment such as a hospital-based antenatal clinic that is apparently midwife-led, the midwives' professional autonomy is still constrained. For example, a midwife is unable to arrange an ultrasound scan for a woman without the obstetrician's authorisation, so although the scan is clinically warranted, the official justification for the procedure must come from the obstetrician. Therefore, although midwives who do not have to rotate are able to consolidate their skills, they still do not have full professional autonomy. However, in this context, it could be argued that those who do have to rotate have restrictions placed on their development by virtue of the fact that they do not have the opportunity to consolidate their skills *and* they face curtailments imposed by obstetric protocols. Indeed, Coyle et al (2001) quoting from McCourt and Page (1996) wonder whether midwife-led care is workable in an obstetric-led unit. As the example of referral for ultrasound illustrates, the midwife's judgement about who really needs to be referred to an obstetrician is restricted. So while a midwife-led antenatal clinic seems to be a step towards normalising pregnancy, this is only an illusion if protocols demand that midwives have to refer routine checks to obstetricians as a matter of course, even if this is not clinically necessary. This can only further undermine midwives' sense of professional autonomy, and also their authority in the eyes of their patients.

But services such as midwife-led care do not have to be organised in this way. As the DoH (2001) report *Shifting the Balance of Power: Securing Delivery* puts it: '[s]taff need to be involved in decisions which affect service delivery. Empowerment comes when staff own the policies and are able to bring about real change' (Department of Health 2001 p 24). This suggests that if midwives are seen as sufficiently professionally autonomous to devise and regulate their own policies, enhanced professional autonomy should follow.

Some midwives would welcome the opportunity to act on the recommendations of *Changing Childbirth*. They may, however, be constrained if their individual NHS Trust is unwilling to implement the new types of care, perhaps because they consider the perceived benefits for women to be unproven or because funding was denied once the initial pilot schemes of care were completed. Therefore, even midwives who support the new types of care may not have the opportunity to implement them. However, there may be grounds for saying that midwives who elected to practise in the new types of care may forfeit a 'lesser' degree of their autonomy than those who were not given the option. Nevertheless, we should guard against over-generalisation and bear in mind that what may be seen as a 'reasonable' degree of autonomy by one midwife could be viewed in a different light by others. Different midwives will judge the respective benefits and disadvantages of the new care types in different ways. For example, a midwife who has been working on the antenatal clinic on a permanent basis is unlikely to welcome enforced rotation, being unwilling to forfeit this specialised 'niche' in the organisation. A recently qualified midwife whose training was undertaken alongside a midwife whose contract was rotational may view the situation differently. It could be said that the recently qualified midwife would be familiar with the idea of rotation in midwifery practice, and so would forfeit less professional autonomy than the antenatal clinic midwife in this instance. Arguably, though, both midwives may be unable to consolidate their new skills.

EFFECTS ON WOMEN

The retention crisis in midwifery has brought about adverse consequences on women's options and the care provided. Fewer practising midwives may result in women receiving less care or care that is inconsistent with their clinical condition. The Royal College of Midwives (1999) concluded that maternity units will be forced to prioritise the range of options they can offer to women. The bottom line here is that it may be more cost effective to accept a higher rate of caesarean sections than to offer women one-to-one support in labour. (There is some evidence suggesting that staffing difficulties are associated with a higher intervention rate (RCM 2000 p 22).) Such policy decisions clearly have an effect on whether or not women can receive the care that they have chosen, and whether their consent to interventions is invalidated by the lack of choice at an earlier stage. Most women will agree to necessary interventions, but what becomes necessary may be caused not by any underlying condition or factors in their pregnancy, but by the kind of care they received leading up to the crisis that required intervention.

Staff are an important resource. If midwifery staffing levels remain critically low, women-centred schemes such as early labour assessments at home, domiciliary fetal monitorings and community-based drop-in clinics may not be available because the midwives allocated to provide them have conflicting and overriding responsibilities elsewhere. Moreover, given the current climate, it is difficult to see how midwives can promote women's autonomy within reasonable boundaries when their own professional autonomy is curtailed. In this sense both women and midwives are casualties in the current system.

The RCM (2000) drew on research by the Economic and Social Research Council (ESRC) that showed one of the consequences of the retention crisis to be that staffing shortages have led to the cancellation of antenatal and postnatal visits, thus limiting the opportunities for midwives to provide this care (RCM 2000 p 20). It is a moot point whether less care in this context is a bad thing. Sometimes routine care results from traditional practice rather than clinical need. Where this is the case, then the midwife's time could actually be better spent elsewhere. Less monitoring of normal pregnancies might mark a shift away from the medicalisation of pregnancy, which in its turn may actually facilitate greater choice for women who want a more natural pregnancy and childbirth experience.

This shift may, however, ignore the psychosocial aspects of midwifery care that are more difficult to measure and assess. If women have less contact with midwives they lose the opportunity to discuss a wide range of concerns, including the kind of delivery that they might prefer, and also to discuss the delivery that they did have, which might not have gone as they had hoped. For instance, it can be therapeutic for women who have had an unexpected though necessary instrumental delivery to talk to a midwife about this, and it may take some coming to terms with even though the overall result—a healthy mother and baby—was good. If staffing levels are low, at worst, the woman may never receive this postnatal debriefing and at best it may be no more than a 'narrative' of events reiterated by the professional. Sometimes what women need is a more personalised account of events and not one that could have been given to any woman in her position. This is also part of what it means to promote woman-centred care.

CONCLUSION

In the light of the current retention crisis, there may be grounds for saying that midwives should reappraise their role. Midwives need to regulate their own professional affairs and practise as midwives should. What is needed is more than a change in the organisation of service provision. One way of achieving this reappraisal might be for midwives and their managers to collectively exercise their professional autonomy to create care options that should ultimately benefit women. Midwives need to reclaim their role as experts in normal midwifery practice.

It is virtually certain that midwives will never be 'fully' professionally autonomous and the search for renewed autonomy must be confined within reasonable ethical boundaries. Greater professional control should not be gained at the price of diminished autonomy for pregnant women. In keeping the balance we must bear in mind that workload pressures could exacerbate the current retention crisis in midwifery. Woman-centred care can only be undermined by deteriorating staffing levels that influence the quality of care women receive. Developmental support needs to become a key feature of the new schema of care. In the early days of any innovation, it may be difficult to assess the level of expertise needed across the range of midwifery practice, but evaluation must extend to the sustainability of the new schemes of care being implemented. Collectively, these could be seen as 'quality' issues that in turn influence the type of care women receive.

References

Ball L, Curtis P, Kirkham M 2002 Why do midwives leave? RCM, London
Barbour L 2001 RCOG–RCM a marriage made in heaven? The Practising Midwife 4(7):41–43
Beauchamp T L, Childress J F 1994 Principles of biomedical ethics, 4th edn. Oxford University Press, Oxford
Bradshaw G, Bradshaw P L 1997 The professionalisation of midwifery. Modern Midwife 7(12):23–26
Coyle K, Hauck Y, Percival P et al 2001 Normality and collaboration: mothers' perceptions on birth centre versus hospital care. Midwifery 17:182–193
Department of Health 1993 Changing childbirth: report of the Expert Maternity Group. HMSO, London
Department of Health 1999 Making a difference: strengthening the nursing, midwifery and health visiting contribution to health and health care. Department of Health, London
Department of Health 2001 Shifting the balance of power: securing delivery. Department of Health, London
English National Board 1995 Control in practice: to meet the challenge of Changing Childbirth midwifery education resource pack. ENB, London
Harcombe J 1999 Power and political power positions in maternity care. British Journal of Midwifery 7(2):78–82

Harrison S, Pollitt S 1994 Controlling health professionals: the future of work and organisation in the National Health Service. Open University Press, Milton Keynes

Kirkham M J 1999 The culture of midwifery in the National Health Service in England. Journal of Advanced Nursing 30(3):732–739

McCourt C, Page L (eds) 1996 Report on the evaluation of one-to-one midwifery. Thames Valley University, London

O'Dowd A 2000 Midwives need a carrot to return to the NHS. Nursing Times 96(37):5

Royal College of Midwives (RCM) 1999 Evidence to the review body for nursing staff, midwives, health visitors and professions allied to medicine for 2000. RCM, London

Royal College of Midwives (RCM) 2000 Evidence to the review body for nursing staff, midwives, health visitors and professions allied to medicine for 2001. RCM, London

Royal College of Midwives (RCM) 2002 Evidence to the review body for nursing staff, midwives, health visitors and professions allied to medicine for 2003. RCM, London

Shallow H 2001 Competence and confidence: working in a climate of fear. British Journal of Midwifery 9(4):237–244

Stafford S 2001 Lack of autonomy: a reason for midwives leaving the profession? The Practising Midwife 4(7):46–47

Symon A 1996 Midwives and professional status. British Journal of Midwifery 4(10):543–550

United Kingdom Central Council for Nursing, Midwifery and Health Visiting 1992 Code of professional conduct. UKCC, London

United Kingdom Central Council for Nursing, Midwifery and Health Visiting 1998 Midwives rules and code of practice. UKCC, London

Walsh D 2000 Part four fetal monitoring should be controlled. British Journal of Midwifery 8(8):511–516

Chapter **14**

Midwifery research: some ethical considerations

Carolyn Hicks

INTRODUCTION

Over the last few years increasing pressure has been directed at health care professionals to extend the research base of their practice (Department of Health 1993, Peckham 1991). The reason underpinning these moves stems from the current emphasis on public accountability—it is no longer considered acceptable for health care delivery to be founded on traditional and historical precedent rather than sound empirical evidence. Moreover, the need for cost-effective clinical provision in an era which combines diminishing resources with a growing demand for high quality health care, have together made it necessary for all health care professionals to ensure that their practice is founded on the best available research evidence. It has been estimated that up to a billion pounds could be released by withdrawing from unnecessary and ineffective treatments (New & Le Grand 1996). It is hardly surprising, therefore, that huge investments have been made at national and local levels to ensure that not only is sound research being conducted in every clinical arena, but also that the results are being implemented in practice. As a consequence the paramedical professions are being urged to conduct research within their own areas of responsibility in order to challenge existing practices, to identify cost-effective interventions and, through these activities, to enhance the quality of care.

Within midwifery, the importance of research to practice is reflected in the International Code of Ethics for Midwives (International Confederation of Midwives 1993) which states that midwives should, 'develop and share midwifery knowledge through a variety of processes such as peer review and research'. One consequence of these various directives and initiatives has been an expansion of midwifery research that not only challenges the assumptions of existing practices (Brown et al 1999, Ireland et al 2000, Mosley et al 2001), but also evaluates the impact of innovative schemes and government policy on care (McCourt & Pearce 2000, Sheehan 1999, Spurgeon et al 2001). The increasing pressure on journal space and the burgeoning of relevant journals are further testimony to the evidence-based health care culture that is being embraced by a growing proportion of midwives. Indeed, Renfrew's (2000) review of midwifery research recorded on the MIRIAD database notes that in the 5-year period between 1974 and 1979, there were just 17 studies, compared with 219 for the 5 years between 1990 and 1994. It might reasonably be inferred, then, that the potential for ethical problems might rise in direct proportion to the amount of research being conducted.

Although ethical considerations should be the governing principle of any research, the issue is particularly compounded by the current obsession with the randomised controlled trial (RCT) as the gold standard for health care research. The various centres for the systematic review and dissemination of research, such as the Cochrane collaboration, focus almost exclusively on published research which uses RCTs. Consequently, implementation of new models of care often rely on results from RCTs, or a meta-analysis of RCTs in a particular area (e.g. Waldenstrom & Turnbull's 1998 systematic review comparing continuity of midwifery care with standard maternity services). Given that the RCT methodology was originally developed for use in horticulture, where ethical problems are considerably fewer, it follows that the essential design principles of RCTs may be wholly inappropriate for human subjects. Yet because RCTs carry such kudos, the likelihood of obtaining funding and having research results published is increased when this methodology is adopted (Black 1996). As a result, there is an undoubted incentive to adopt the RCT paradigm, even when it may be inappropriate. Yet there are ethical difficulties generated by RCT research that require special consideration. An overview of some of the major considerations is presented in a separate section later in this chapter.

Acknowledgement of the importance of research-based practice is reflected in the changes to the core curriculum of midwifery training courses, many of which incorporate research skills. This, together with a shift in health care culture towards evidence-based clinical service, means that many midwives, newly equipped with the necessary skills, are embarking on research activities at some level. But because midwifery research has as a principal focus of its activities some of the most vulnerable sectors of the population—fetuses, neonates, women in pain or distress—midwives, almost more than many other professional groups, have a particular responsibility to those who participate in their research. Renfrew (2000) in the review noted earlier, however, found that only 60% of researchers had sought research ethics committee (REC) approval for their studies. It was also clear that many of those studies that had not been submitted for REC approval should have been. Ethical issues pervade every aspect of research, from the initial decision to conduct the project, through the choice of design and participants, to the means of disseminating the results. Midwife-researchers must recognise their responsibilities by ensuring that they are fully aware of the ethical principles that guide research. This chapter is an attempt to bring together the most important of these considerations as they apply to midwifery research. Further, more detailed information is available in Eckstein's (2003) text and on the following websites: http://www.corec.org.uk; http:// doh.gov.uk/research/rd3/nhsrandd/researchgovernance.

ETHICAL ISSUES IN RESEARCH

The overriding concern of any researcher using human subjects must be the protection of their rights, dignity and physical and psychological welfare. Any activity that compromises the interests of participants is ethically suspect. Indeed, the Declaration of Helsinki (World Health Organisation 2000) insists that 'the interest of science and society should never take precedence over considerations related to the well-being of the subject'. Consequently, the rights of individuals must be protected. To this end every health authority is required to set up a Local Research Ethics Committee (LREC), the remit of which is to assess proposed research, to ensure that it is ethical and that the potential participants are fully and properly protected. It is essential, then, that for the protection of both researcher and research participants ethical approval is sought and obtained for all projects.

The International Council of Nurses (ICN 1996) outlines six key principles that should guide the research of nurses and midwives. These are:

1. *Beneficence.* The research should benefit both the participant and the wider community through the acquisition of new knowledge. In practice this means that the individual who consents to take part in the research will not only receive additional attention, but may also receive treatment interventions that non-participants cannot access.

2. *Non-maleficence.* Research should cause neither physical nor psychological harm to the participants.

3. *Confidentiality.* The confidentiality of any data provided by participants in a research project must be respected. The identification of the individual or the institution must be protected. Confidential information can only be disclosed with the permission of participants, and not just the doctors or health professionals involved in their care.

4. *Justice.* All participants must be treated fairly and without preference. It is ethically dubious to provide a treatment intervention for some participants and not for others, especially if non-treatment may be a disadvantage.

5. *Fidelity.* When conducting research, a relationship must be built between the participant and the researcher such that the researcher takes responsibility for the welfare of all the participants. This trust is crucial to the research, since it provides protection from risk.

6. *Veracity.* In order to develop the bond identified above, the researcher must not deceive or trick the participant in any way. Withholding information can be as deceitful as the commission of an untruth.

These six guiding principles can be distilled into four rights: the right not to be harmed; the right of privacy, confidentiality and anonymity; the right of self-determination (i.e. the choice of whether to participate, not to participate or to withdraw from the study at any time, without compromising care); and the right of full disclosure (ICN, 1996). These are cardinal rules and will be referred to throughout the rest of the chapter.

These principles clearly need to be translated into practice and it is the aim of this chapter to show how they might be applied in research practice. To this end, the chapter is structured around the following questions:

- What is the research topic?
- Who is to conduct the research?
- Who will benefit from the research?
- Where will the research be conducted?
- How will the participants be treated?
- How will the research be carried out?
- How will the findings be disseminated?

The ethical considerations inherent to every question will be considered separately.

WHAT IS THE RESEARCH TOPIC?

Research is about asking questions and finding answers to those questions in a systematic and objective way. However, the sort of research question being asked may raise a number of ethical issues at the outset that have to be balanced against the anticipated benefits of the research. The issues of beneficence and non-maleficence are crucial here.

All research should start with the assumption it will have some value to someone. Research for its own sake is unlikely to be sanctioned by ethical committees, especially where human participation is involved. Thus any proposed midwifery intervention that has no theoretical or experiential support for its potential usefulness should be rejected. Moreover resources should not be wasted on pointless exercises unlikely to contribute to the corpus of midwifery knowledge.

Many research topics are inherently controversial and potentially very damaging. Investigations into racial differences inevitably raise objections, in part because the findings can be misrepresented as a means of introducing discriminatory and abusive practices. Research that probes into embarrassing or intimate aspects of a participant's experience also requires particular justification, since it will almost certainly cause distress and anxiety. Midwifery research may frequently be involved with private aspects of an individual's behaviour and lifestyle, such as sexual behaviour, drug use, HIV, and so on. For example, Whelan & Lupton (1998) conducted a study of breast-feeding practices among unemployed women and those who were on state benefits without first obtaining REC approval. The implications for these socially disadvantaged women and the mechanism by which the potentially sensitive information regarding income was obtained caused concern, particularly with regard to confidentiality (McHaffie 1998). This is not to suggest that research concerning these topics should be abandoned, but rather that a careful cost–benefit analysis should be undertaken, so that the potential advantages of the research can be weighed against the disadvantages to the participants. If the midwife-researcher decides that the potential benefits outweigh the potential harms, then the research methodology selected must reflect the sensitive nature of the research question using only those procedures that will minimise participant distress.

WHO IS TO CONDUCT THE RESEARCH?

Good research is only possible if there is mutual respect and confidence between the researcher and the participant (see the fidelity and veracity principles). Therefore, anybody who conducts research, especially that which involves human subjects, must be skilled, competent and able to do so. Midwife-researchers should, therefore, take responsibility for ensuring that their understanding of research procedures in the very widest sense is as full and comprehensive as possible. Where the responsibility for the research is shared, then any midwife who observes a co-researcher acting incompetently or engaging in practices that are contrary to ethical conduct, must be prepared to take appropriate action. This poses potential difficulties, particularly if the offending co-worker is senior to the midwife. However, the overriding consideration must always be the welfare of the research participants and anything that threatens this must be stopped. Failure or refusal to accept responsibility for co-workers is itself a potential ethical problem.

Related to this is the issue of sponsored research. Science is supposed to be objective and independent, but this position may be undermined if an organisation or company that has a vested interest in the outcome finances the research. Renfrew's report on the MIRIAD database indicates that 86% of all the midwifery research entered had been funded and, of this, 46 (18%) of the studies had received support from commercial sponsors. Where the researchers are paid employees of such a company, their objectivity in the research may be influenced by their dependency on the company for a job. This is not to suggest dishonesty but merely that the freedom of the researcher to design an objective piece of research and report and publish all the salient findings might be limited by the company's need to present their product to potential customers in the most seductive and enticing light (Morin et al 2002, Office of the Inspector General 2000). It is indeed well known within medical circles that there have been many instances in the past where adverse results have been suppressed in order to safeguard the product under investigation. The Thalidomide scandal (Sjostrom and Nilsson 1972) is perhaps the most obvious example. Indeed, as Morin et al (2002) note, such is the relentless pressure on pharmaceutical companies to produce new drugs that clinical research has become a natural breeding ground for sins of omission and commission. Such control over the research, and the motivations underlying this control, constitute a very serious ethical problem for many researchers, particularly in times when alternative employment may be hard to find and fixed-term contracts are the norm. Therefore, the role and position of the researcher is a critical one. In an ideal world, researchers are competent, autonomous and independent; in reality, they may be 'the hired hand doing the bidding of the paymaster ... or ... simply an ammunition wagon, loaded with powerful knowledge just waiting to be used, whether the users are the "good guys" or "the bad guys"' (Robson 1993 p 01).

The investigator is not always the one in a relatively weak position, however, and is commonly in a position of influence and authority over the participants—particularly in medically related research when a clear dominant–subordinate relationship normally exists between the health care professional and the patient. In these circumstances, patients/clients may feel under an obligation to the researcher and so may comply with research demands simply to ensure that they will not be disadvantaged in other aspects of their care. This places enormous responsibilities on researchers to ensure they do not abuse their position of authority either to coerce patients to participate/ remain within the project or to influence the participants' responses in a way that benefits the research (see the fidelity principle). If the researcher cannot guarantee that these malpractices will not occur then it is essential that a disinterested colleague who is not directly responsible for the research or patient's care conducts the study and/or recruitment of participants. Under these conditions it is easier for the patient/client to withdraw from the study.

WHO WILL BENEFIT FROM THE RESEARCH?

The question of who will benefit from the research may well give rise to grandiose, if somewhat naive, answers of 'humanity' and 'medical science' and subsume the concepts of beneficence and non-malefi-cance. More realistically, it is likely that only a small subgroup of the population will derive any short- or long-term good. For example, Wilkund et al (2000) investigated the experiences of nine Somali women giving birth in Sweden, and seven partners. While this has clear relevance for other Somali families in the country, it does not generalise much beyond this small cohort. This does not invalidate the research by any means, but it is important that the beneficiaries of the study are honestly identified. The reason for this relates back to the point about who conducts the research. If the investigator is a paid employee of a large corporation—for instance an infant food manufacturer—then it is quite conceivable that the principal benefi-ciary may be the sponsor, especially if restrictions are imposed regarding the nature, conduct and publication of the research. Benefits may also accrue to the researchers who, if they provide their employer with the desired results, may have their contracts extended. The implicit cynicism in this message is becoming an increasing reality now that the public service sector generally relies more and more heavily on private companies rather than on government departments for its research money.

The benefits of an active research profile are also evident within higher education. The obsession in the university sector with published research means that one route to a meteoric career in academia is through the relentless publication of research in peer-reviewed journals. This has obvious implications for those midwives who are employed wholly or partly within the tertiary education sector, since promotion will be heavily dependent on research productivity. The temptation to churn out research that has not been thoroughly scrutinised for its ethical acceptability is a serious problem.

Even if the midwife is an independent and autonomous researcher, it is still conceivable that the benefits accruing from the research will be greater for the investigator than for the investigated. Research carries considerable kudos in most professional domains and consequently any researchers who generate a set of interesting results may enhance their prestige and even career prospects. With so many potential vested interests in play, it is important that potential benefits that might accrue to the investigator, the sponsor, or even to the knowledge base of midwifery must be very carefully and honestly acknowledged so that they are not allowed to bias the nature and conduct of the project and its impact on the participants. Polit & Hungler (1995) provide a useful overview of the risk–benefit ratio in health research.

WHERE WILL THE RESEARCH BE CONDUCTED?

Working on the assumption that midwifery research has the potential to improve client well-being and care, the question of where to conduct the research must, of necessity, raise key ethical considerations, since participating venues may have a potential advantage over those units not selected for study.

Conversely, the selection of a particular venue for the research may fuel an already explosive situation, simply by its focus of attention; for example, a hypothetical study conducted in a large urban psychiatric unit might have found that additional resources were earmarked for and directed to managing postpartum depression in an ethnic minority, and in a resource-strapped area of provision, any inequalities, whether intentional or accidental, might inflame local tension and discrimination. While any set of research findings has the potential to be misused, for politically sensitive topics the dissemination of results in a public arena may trigger adverse reactions, especially if the locus of the research in identifiable. Alternatively, targeting particular geographical areas for health education literature on smoking and alcohol use during pregnancy might inadvertently suggest that some social classes are more likely to harm the fetus in these ways. While the design of any study that used non-representative sampling may be questionable, the reality is that much published research is small-scale, locally funded and locally conducted, which may mean that convenience samples are used rather than a more valid sampling frame. Once again, whatever the potential for difficulty, it must be weighed against the wider value of the information that can be gained from the project.

There is one further point regarding the selection of a research venue. Many units are more than happy to cooperate with research activities simply because there will be tangible gains for them, at least in the short term. One example of this might be the (temporary) provision of an ultrasound scanner in a remote rural health centre, in order to look at its impact on early identification of fetal abnormality in a population too distant from the main hospital to take advantage of its services. For the duration of the project, the centre, at no cost to itself, would have additional screening resources. The provision of additional staff, equipment and even drugs is arguably a necessary aspect of research, for it would be wrong for research to place additional burdens on an already overstretched service. Clearly, such additional resources are likely to be welcomed by the unit receiving them; however, these additional resources might act as an inducement to a unit to participate. Even if no technical equipment goes with participation, it is quite likely that the researcher might constitute an extra pair of hands or other resource. Ironically, while patients are protected from financial coercion or inducement, units are not. Clearly, then, the wider implications of a research project must be considered fully. All trials inevitably come to an end, which may leave participating units with reduced resources and raised patient expectations of enhanced service provision. Clearly, this is not a sufficient reason to stop the termination of the research activity, but it does highlight the importance of keeping all research participants fully informed about the impact and implications of the study, before, during and on its conclusion.

HOW WILL THE PARTICIPANTS BE TREATED?

The research participants are the cornerstone of any study and the protection of their rights, dignity and well-being must be the primary concern of the researcher, as outlined in the six principles above. Indeed, the major responsibility of any REC is to ensure that the subjects are treated in a way that does not compromise their mental and physical welfare. Although the protection of research participants' welfare is an obvious primary consideration, there are numerous examples from the annals of health research that suggest that the abuse of participants is far from uncommon. One of the most appalling examples was the Tuskegee Study of Untreated Syphilis (Brawley 1999, Gamble 1997). In essence, this study withheld treatment for syphilis from 399 black males from a poor socioeconomic background and monitored the effects. The men had no idea that there was an effective intervention available, nor were they informed about the consequences of non-treatment. At first glance this study appears to have little relevance for midwifery; however, its ramifications for women's health (Gamble 1997), involvement of minority groups in research (Brawley 1999, Corbie-Smith et al 1999) and public confidence in research (Corbie-Smith et al 1999) have been enormous and clearly demonstrate the wide-ranging implications of ethically bankrupt research protocols. This study breached all six of the guiding principles for ethical research, and as a result not only compromised the participants but also the wider research agenda. Treatment of the participants is heavily bound up with the type of methodology adopted in the study and this is dealt with in the next section.

The main focus of the World Medical Association's Declaration of Helsinki (World Health Organisation 2000) is the protection of the research participants, whose welfare must take priority over the interests of the wider scientific community and the public. Particular attention is directed at vulnerable groups, especially those who cannot give consent for themselves (babies and fetuses are obviously relevant here), those who will not benefit personally from the research and those for whom the research is integral to their care. There is a clearly stated obligation to protect the life, health, dignity and privacy of the participants. Similarly, research guidelines of the ICN (1996), the British Psychological Society (2000) and the American Psychological Association (2002) are concerned with the welfare of the participants, and any intending midwife researcher should study these documents in detail. In midwifery research, these concerns are heightened because of the vulnerability of the likely research participants. The particular ethical problems associated with midwifery research relate to the issue of consent, which requires the participants' competent, voluntary and informed agreement to take part in the research. Obviously, in the case of a baby, embryo or fetus, it is the parents who are asked for their agreement and while this is the logical and proper alternative it does nonetheless raise special concerns among research ethics committees and researchers.

Gaining proper consent is a fundamental aspect of ethically acceptable research. Every risk involved in the research must be properly explained and understood. In addition, the procedures involved must be described fully where possible, but this in itself may provoke debate. Many studies, for example, would be rendered valueless if the intentions and methods were outlined to participants beforehand, simply because advance knowledge may create a set of expectations in the participants which may distort the outcome. For example Hicks (1992) investigated how a sample of clinical midwives viewed research conducted by midwives as opposed to that carried out by doctors. Two articles on the same midwifery topic were distributed to the group. However, half the group were told that the research for the first article had been conducted by a midwife and the second by a doctor, while for the rest of the group, the information was reversed. The midwives were asked to read both articles and then to evaluate them according to a number of specified criteria. The articles allegedly conducted by the midwife were evaluated significantly lower on a number of key criteria than the articles purported to have been carried out by the doctor. The methodology here could legitimately be criticised for its duplicity, since the participants were deceived regarding the authorship of the papers. However, it is obvious that had the group been informed of the true authorship in advance of the study, then the results would have been invalid. Many other examples abound where the methodology involves deceiving the participants in some way as a necessary expedient of a valid research design. Studies that involve placebos, for example, are good illustrations of necessary duplicity (though this can be limited by telling all the participants that some of them may be randomly allocated a placebo). If participants were told in advance that they were receiving an inactive therapy, it would be virtually impossible to measure the placebo effect accurately. The favoured RCT paradigm depends heavily on placebos, non-treatment groups and participants' lack of knowledge regarding the nature of their own treatment intervention and consequently raises serious ethical questions. This will be discussed in more detail in the section on RCTs.

While deception may be an unavoidable aspect of the methodology it is not necessarily desirable, since tricking innocent participants in this way cannot conceivably be regarded as ethically ideal. However, as Coolican (1992) implies there may be no methodologically acceptable alternative. The resolution of this problem again revolves around a full cost–benefit analysis—do the anticipated benefits of the study outweigh the disadvantages of the design, and can the deception be minimised in some way, such as informing all participants that they could potentially receive a placebo? (See Polit & Hungler 1995 for a fuller discussion.)

Whatever the level of deception, however, it is imperative that the researcher debriefs the participants at the conclusion of the project. The debriefing must reveal the real purpose and aims of the project and, very importantly, must ensure that the participants feel the same about themselves when they leave as they did when they arrived. Stanley Milgram's (1963, 1974) seminal study of obedience to authority is a classic example of how the deception that was necessary to undertake the study had a very negative impact on participants' subsequent self-perceptions and self-beliefs. While this study may seem far removed from midwifery research, a similarly duplicitous follow-up in a hospital revealed shocking levels of unquestioning compliance to authority by nursing staff, which, despite debriefing, had an adverse impact on the self-image of the participating nurses (Hofling et al 1966). The point here is that to preserve an individual's dignity there may be some circumstances that require the investigator to modify the feedback to participants. Where the midwife-researcher is uncertain about the nature and extent of any duplicitous procedures used, then advice should be sought from experienced and impartial colleagues who have no investment in the study's outcomes. The role of RECs is also important in these circumstances, where the central guiding principle is always the minimisation of any potential short-, medium- or long-term mental and physical distress for the participants.

In health research, there are also the possible problems surrounding the use of new treatments with side-effects that are unknown, of denying someone a treatment that has demonstrable value or of using overly intrusive techniques. While these issues are fundamentally methodological in nature, they do have implications for participant welfare. Lest the reader should protest that such issues are well outside the province of midwifery research, some illustrations may be useful. As an illustration of the first point, take a project whose focus is the use of a specially designed exercise programme intended to invert known breech presentations to cephalic presentations. It seems innocuous enough but the procedure would involve selecting a group of women and asking them to comply with an exercise régime assumed (at least theoretically), to be useful, but without any evidence as to its value. Could it lead to adverse side-effects? With regard to the second point, treatment may be withheld in some studies that use a control group; for example, if the midwife was interested in assessing the benefits of counselling for women who have delivered babies with an impairment, it would be necessary to look at comparable women who received no such support. Is it ethical to withhold this intervention? Dilemmas such as this have led to the introduction of more stringent codes of practice, which encourage the control group to be given the *standard* form of treatment against which a comparison with the trial group can be made. However, since the original definition of the control group was as a non-intervention group, these modifications should be regarded as an expedient adopted to resolve the tension between the need for scientific rigour and ethical probity. This issue is discussed more fully in the next section. The third point regarding the use of overly intrusive techniques can be illustrated by the use of questionnaires that investigate the respondent's previous or current sexual activities, illegal substance use, and so on. The large body of evidence that has been amassed on the evaluation of the 'changing childbirth' initiative, for example, also illustrates each of these points (North Staffordshire Changing Childbirth Research Team 2000, Spurgeon et al 2001, Hicks et al 2003). While it was assumed from the outset that midwifery-led care would be beneficial to maternal well-being, because it was untested there was still the possibility of risk to babies, mothers and even the midwives themselves. Allocation of women to traditional care or midwifery-led care also meant that one group might have had compromised outcomes and a lower quality of service provision. Each of these examples illustrates the particular problems that health researchers face when attempting to find a compromise position between ethical and scientific acceptability.

Sometimes the research methodology involves the observation of participants in naturalistic settings. However if subjects are aware that they are being watched, it is highly likely that their behaviour will change significantly, thereby undermining the naturalistic nature of the study. Consequently, participants may be observed without being aware of it. This may be considered an invasion of privacy, even when the behaviour seems innocent, but it is undoubtedly unacceptable if private and personal behaviours are under scrutiny. Consider, for example, a study that looks at the responses of a woman and her partner to a male midwife who assists during the second stage of labour. It is conceivable that the investigator might record a number of verbal and non-verbal responses in the couple when a shift change results in the arrival of a male midwife. The situation might be observed via a one-way mirror (a very typical way of conducting an observational study), which would enable the investigator to conduct the study without being seen and therefore without any of the participants being aware of what was going on. Such an 'intrusion' into a very private and personal event without prior permission is a serious contravention of ethical codes of conduct. And yet, the available evidence suggests that not only is it essential that naturalistic events are recorded without participants' knowledge, since awareness will distort the behaviour, but also there again appears to be no satisfactory methodological alternative (Coolican, 1992). As with other ethical issues arising out of the conflict between sound methodology and ethical acceptability, it is important that any studies involving non-voluntary participation are discussed with colleagues who are experienced in research matters.

Generally, however, the British Psychological Society's Ethical Guidelines (2000) suggest that observational research is only acceptable in those situations when the participants would normally expect to be observed by strangers, and also that due consideration should be taken with respect to cultural and local mores and values since it is easy to infringe these quite unwittingly.

It is good practice to ensure that any research procedure likely to cause distress of any sort should use the minimum possible number of participants. This is contrary to the common perception that the greater the number of subjects the better the study. This is a myth that is neither valid from a methodological viewpoint nor acceptable from an ethical one. While it is clear that there must be a mid-position between sound research procedures and ethical considerations, the potential impact on the participants must always be a primary concern.

Where some discomfort is inevitable, the researcher must recognise the right of the participants to refuse to participate. In order to exercise that right though, the participants must be fully informed about the risks and their right to withdraw from the research at any point and for whatever reason. There may also be situations when the investigator decides to terminate the study because the observed problems are greater than anticipated.

Particular difficulties arise when participants are paid or remunerated in some way for their participation (Harries & Edwards 1994). This situation can create an employer/employee relationship with an implicit contractual obligation. In these instances, the 'employer' may feel empowered to make excessive or unreasonable demands of the 'employee', who, in turn, may feel obliged to tolerate unacceptable procedures or produce the responses desired by the 'employer' but which may not be their honest reactions. While payment of subjects may invalidate consent, Morin et al (2002) have noted that in the US, many pharmaceutical companies allow between $2000 and $5000 per recruit to drugs trials. Likewise, in the UK, Foy et al (1998) found that GPs are frequently offered substantial sums of money or its equivalent for each patient recruited into a clinical trial.

The need to protect the privacy and confidentiality of subjects is a key issue in all research. All participants have the right to anonymity, privacy and confidentiality and if this cannot be guaranteed, then the participant must be informed immediately and given the right to withdraw from the project. Any participant who has been deceived about this point has the right to witness the destruction of any data and information concerning them (Data Protection Act 1998). There may also be a case for litigation. However, sometimes the investigator may wish to follow up individual cases, which is impossible if anonymity is absolute. In these cases, the researcher may eliminate any identification of the individual by name, but instead may use a numerical or alphabetic code. In this way the privacy of the individual is maintained while allowing for possible follow-up by the researcher.

The issue of confidentiality, while a crucial one, generates its own problems. If participants have performed particularly well, honourably or diligently during a project, is it not reasonable that they should be rewarded? For example, an anonymous survey of working practices among community midwives might reveal a small cohort who routinely operate over and above the call of duty, not only in terms of the hours worked, but also in the tasks undertaken and the results obtained. There is a cogent argument that they should have just reward, but this is clearly impossible if the study conforms to the confidentiality rule. Conversely, if the survey found that a small number of community midwives were behaving negligently or improperly, then the protection of their identity also serves to perpetuate their malpractice. Or suppose a researcher found that a midwife or client had undisclosed HIV, and that they were putting at risk many of those with whom they came into close contact. In both cases, disclosure might be in the public interest and indeed may arguably be required by professional codes of conduct.

During research—particularly that in the health care arena—it is quite likely that the researcher may come across a problem of which the participant is unaware. In such circumstances, it is the responsibility of the researcher to inform the participant of this problem if it is believed that by withholding this information the participant's well-being may be compromised. Understandably, once aware of this problem the participant may seek the advice of the researcher. Only if the researcher is fully qualified should this advice be proffered, otherwise the appropriate professional help should be facilitated.

HOW WILL THE RESEARCH BE CARRIED OUT?

Research involves midwives asking questions about their practice or observations and then using scientific methods to answer those questions. There are two basic research methodologies available to the midwife-researcher, each of which stems from a different set of assumptions. These methodologies are called *qualitative* and *quantitative* methods.

Qualitative research

Qualitative research involves the naturalistic study of the client/patient as a whole person (as opposed to a set of behaviours or symptoms) within a social framework. The researcher attempts to gain insight into the client/patient's subjective thoughts, feelings and experiences within a given set of circumstances. Such an approach to midwifery research is common, and indeed, Lydon-Rochelle & Albers (1993) in a survey conducted over 5 years found that 67% of midwifery research used a descriptive/interpretive approach to data collection and analysis. This was confirmed by Renfrew's (2000) analysis of the MIRIAD database. For example, Melender & Lauri (1999) used an interview approach to investigate the fears concerning pregnancy and childbirth in women who had recently given birth. The researchers carried out the study within 2–3 days post-delivery. To conduct this research, they were in close personal interaction with the mothers, recording their descriptions of their reactions to pregnancy and birth. From these descriptions, they gained insight into the highly personal and subjective experience of giving birth. The researchers discussed their interpretations of the interview data in order to identify common themes. The value of this study is primarily in the enhanced understanding of the fears and anxieties that women may have about the pregnancy and birth experience, so that health care delivery in this context can be modified to improve the client's experiences. It is worth emphasising, however, that qualitative research paradigms are frequently used to elicit personal feelings and experiences and this inevitably may mean that there is some intrusion into the participants' privacy. The researcher, having obtained informed consent, must therefore be careful to preserve the confidentiality of the data.

Another reason for the popularity of qualitative approaches relates to the fact that it is, by definition, normalistic. This means that there is no manipulation of treatment procedures, no intervention in the service delivery and no withholding of therapy or care. Consequently, there may well be fewer ethical problems that arise. However, any study that focuses on the most intimate thoughts and experiences of an individual must have a fundamental regard for their privacy and well-being. The very content of the interview or questionnaire might be distressing and therefore the participants must always be aware of their right not to participate without fear that their refusal might compromise their care. Moreover, the close relationship that qualitative research requires between the participant and researcher means that objective interpretation of events might be very difficult to achieve. In consequence, bias might creep into the conclusions, with a possible deleterious impact on subsequent health care. To illustrate this, take the example of the quality of care for lesbian mothers. It has been noted (Wilton 1999) that homophobia among midwives compromises the quality of care provided for lesbian mothers. The interrelationship between reproduction and heterosexuality is an obvious one and any variation on this may have specific implications for midwives. It is hardly surprising then, that Wilton found evidence of strongly held views on the topic. Consequently, any midwife-researchers who conduct research in this area may be driven by their own attitudes and beliefs about sexuality. With the best will in the world, it would be difficult for the midwife-researchers to start the project on neutral territory, and so the potential for misinterpreting events as a result of their attitudinal position and expectations is likely to be high. This is not to suggest that the researcher intends to distort the evidence, but rather that the human element which adds richness to the qualitative approach may also detract from the objectivity of the recordings. In such a study, any statement or viewpoint the interviewee proffers that accords with what the researcher expects or hopes to hear may be overemphasised in the report. Conversely, any disclosure that disagrees with the researcher's expectations may be underreported. Consequently, the findings from studies that deal with emotive topics may be vulnerable to some level of distortion of reality. Improvements in objectivity might be achieved by having additional researchers present, so that some counterbalancing of bias and view can be achieved, or alternatively a totally independent, unconnected researcher who has no vested interest in the outcome of the study could be used.

Other methodological problems are associated with qualitative research. The impact of an observer on the participants' behaviour, for example, has already been discussed. In addition, there are difficulties associated with attempting to procure returns in questionnaire surveys. The initial number of returns may often be too low to be of any value and so the researcher sends out reminders to the non-returners. But is this a form of harassment? Many people feel intimidated by this sort of pressure and while a good return rate may be highly desirable from the researcher's perspective, the individual cost to the recipients of written or telephone reminders might be unacceptably high, particularly if the recipient is already vulnerable. Furthermore, there is always the possibility that using normalistic techniques to collect data may reveal health care practices that are unsafe or dangerous. For example, video recording of care practices may demonstrate serious deficiencies in care delivery, which may lead to litigation, or managerial and political manipulation. It is hardly surprising, then, that many health care professionals are very reluctant to take part in such studies. For more information on ethical issues associated with qualitative research, the reader is referred to Parahoo (1997).

Quantitative research

The second major methodological approach is the quantitative method, which as its name suggests involves the collection and analysis of numerical data. Such a technique is often anathema to the health care professions whose tradition has been founded on quality and intuition, rather than on formal quantification. However, the focus on evidence-based health care means that experimental methods, and RCTs in particular, are essential to a more systematic and scientific approach to care delivery.

This approach has its roots firmly fixed in the formal experimental method. It involves the objective, detached measurement of events as a means of testing hypotheses. To do this, the researcher has to control the research situation, and manipulate the procedures in order that cause and effect relationships can be identified. Any findings emerging from the study can be used to predict and control future health care delivery. Just reading this synopsis of the scientific method arouses immediate ethical queries. The vocabulary alone ('control', 'manipulate') is indicative that research participants have lost their freedom to choose and this may be a serious contravention of proper ethical codes of conduct. Whether such an approach can ever be justified in midwifery may be the target of legitimate debate. However, the value of this approach in adding to the knowledge base of midwifery is beyond dispute. Questions such as the following examples can be answered by this method:

- Which care approach is best for a given group of clients?
- Which people are most likely to benefit from a particular intervention?
- What is the most likely course of a specified problem?
- Which interventions are most cost-effective?

These are of vital importance if midwifery care is to be systematised and improved. However, the method involved in answering them may raise ethical problems whose gravity may offset any benefits. The use of a hypothetical example may be the best illustration of this point.

A midwife working in the antenatal clinic of a large teaching hospital is interested in looking at the psychological impact of chorionic villus sampling (CVS) on maternal well-being. Her hypothesis is that CVS has a beneficial effect on the maternal psychological state. She decides to select a group of women who have opted for CVS and to assess their psychological state before and after CVS, thus:

A group of women has:

Pre-CVS measure of psychological state	→	CVS	→	Post-CVS measure of psychological state

By comparing the before and after measures of psychological state, the midwife believes that she will be able to determine the impact of CVS. However, a colleague points out that psychological state might have altered anyway, simply as a function of the stage of the pregnancy. Since CVS is typically performed at a point when the woman has begun to adjust to the knowledge of being pregnant it is quite likely that her psychological state would start to improve at around this time and that any changes observed in the group may reflect this rather than the impact of CVS. To get round this, the midwife-researcher decides to add a control group, comprising a group of women at the same stage of pregnancy who do not undergo CVS. The research design now looks like this:

Group 1:

Pre-CVS measure of psychological state	→	CVS	→	Post-CVS measure of psychological state

Group 2 (control):

First measure of psychological state	→	No CVS	→	Second measure of psychological state

If the two groups of women are the same in all respects bar the CVS, then any differences between them at second testing must be the result of the CVS. By using this improved design, the researcher can indeed answer the question regarding the positive impact CVS has on the woman's psychological state. However, the devil's advocate colleague then points out that the group of women who were offered CVS had all belonged to an 'at-risk' category of mothers who had received genetic counselling prior to pregnancy. The group who did not receive CVS had not been drawn from this category and therefore the study was not comparing like with like. The midwife-researcher reconsiders the design and decides to select a second group of women from the at-risk register, but to withhold the option of CVS. This design now compares like with like but also has some very grave ethical problems. Is it acceptable to withhold treatment, intervention or screening from anyone? This problem is a very difficult one indeed and is a characteristic of any study that uses a 'no-treatment' control group in this way. In such cases, a number of expedients can be adopted. One typical option would be a comparison of two interventions rather than a comparison of one intervention with a no-intervention control group. In this example, then, the impact of CVS would be compared with another similar screening procedure (i.e. amniocentesis) to see if one approach was more beneficial psychologically than the other. However, this option is not particularly useful to our hypothetical study, since amniocentesis is carried out at a later stage in pregnancy and therefore, once again, like is not being compared with like. Nonetheless, the use of a second treatment group for the purposes of comparison can be a valuable and ethically more acceptable option than a control group in many studies and should always be considered where the use of a no-treatment group is dubious. Many examples abound in the midwifery research literature that illustrate the use of an alternative or existing treatment technique, instead of a control group (e.g. Mosley et al 2001, Sheehan 1999).

Another alternative to the predicament of the control group would be to use women in the 'at-risk' group who had voluntarily decided not to have CVS. This is a naturalistic choice that does not force women into situations against their wishes. The revised design now uses two groups of women, both at risk from genetic problems and both at a similar stage of pregnancy where one group has elected to have CVS and the other has not. How acceptable is this design now? The devil's advocate could legitimately continue to criticise by pointing out that the group who choose CVS are likely to do so because they expect that the procedure will have some benefit to them psychologically, by providing knowledge either that the fetus is normal or that there is a problem about which a decision must be made. Either way, the group believes knowledge to be a useful and beneficial outcome to the screening. Therefore, in the group that has CVS there is an expectation of benefit that may not be present in the control group, and it is this expectation rather than the actual procedure or its outcome that has the effect. In order to overcome the problem of expectation in a study, placebo groups are often used. This procedure involves giving some participants an entirely worthless intervention to establish whether the participants' expectation of benefit actually produces any change. This precaution is commonly used in drug trials. If a new drug is being tested, patients taking the drug may show an improvement simply because they expect any treatment to benefit them. In order to counteract this problem, some participants are given useless saline injections, or dummy pills to see if they have an effect. The success of the placebo rests on the patients' ignorance of which trial group they are in, and therefore there is an element of deception in the procedure, which may have ethical implications, as previously discussed.

If this design is incorporated into our hypothetical study then a further group of women would have unwittingly to experience a fake vaginal investigation using instruments and procedures comparable to those used during actual CVS. The study now looks like this:

Group 1:

| Pre-CVS assessment of psychological state | → True CVS → | Post-CVS assessment of psychological state |

Group 2:

| Pretest assessment of psychological state | → Fake CVS → | Post-test assessment of psychological state |

Group 3:

| First assessment of psychological state | → No CVS → | Second assessment of psychological state |

Methodologically, the study has been substantially improved, but these improvements have introduced some very serious ethical concerns. Because neither fake nor true CVS procedures can be forced on the women who have decided to have no screening at all (Group 3), to introduce a placebo procedure means that a selection of women who believed they were choosing CVS will unknowingly have to undergo a useless or even risky procedure. This not only raises the debate discussed earlier regarding deception of participants but also puts physical and psychological welfare at risk through the application of a useless investigation. Moreover, how would the researcher decide who should undergo the true CVS and who the fake? Conventional research procedures would suggest that the women are randomly selected for either condition and in this way they would all have an equal chance of receiving the true CVS. Individual access to appropriate treatment must form a central aspect of any debate regarding research methodology involving randomised trials. This hypothetical example obviously presents a fairly extreme position by way of illustration; many studies investigate research questions about which there is genuine uncertainty about the best course of treatment (equipoise). If there is equipoise, then it is not obvious that either group will be advantaged or disadvantaged.

Our hypothetical study shows that perfect research methodology can sometimes only be achieved at the expense of ethical considerations, and vice versa. However, real-world research in whatever domain must achieve an acceptable balance between the validity of the research procedures and adherence to ethical guidelines. Midwifery research, like all other research whose focus is applied, must select a compromise position that recognises the mutual limitations that ethics and methodology impose on each other.

There are, of course, other techniques of research such as correlational designs and single case studies, all of which have their pitfalls. While problems outlined in this section also apply to these designs, the reader might like to look at Polgar & Thomas (1992) for a more detailed discussion of their particular characteristics.

THE RANDOMISED CONTROLLED TRIAL: A SPECIAL CASE FOR ETHICAL CONSIDERATIONS

The RCT is assumed to be the only methodology that has the rigour necessary to inform clinical decision-making (e.g. Sibbald & Roland 1998). Systematic reviews and meta-analyses of RCTs are undertaken by the centres for dissemination of health care research (e.g. the Cochrane Collaboration), and form the principal mechanism through which scientific research is used to change health care practice. Within midwifery research, there are a significant number of studies using RCTs (e.g. Mosley et al 2001, Waldenstrom & Nilsson 1997), and Renfrew's (2000) analysis of 466 studies registered on the MIRIAD database between 1974 and 1998 found that 16 (5%) used RCTs.

In essence, an RCT is a more tightly controlled, stringent version of the experimental design outlined above. It is characterised by the following features:

- It is controlled: participants are divided into groups, each of which receives either no treatment, a placebo, or the standard available therapy.

- It is randomised: participants are allocated randomly to each arm of the trial.

- It uses a double-blind procedure: neither the researcher nor the participants know in which arm they have been placed.

- The groups are matched on critical variables that are thought to impact on the outcome.

- Procedures are standardised: every participant is treated identically, apart from the nature of the actual intervention.

- It may adopt a crossover design, which means that during the course of the research, groups are reassigned to a different treatment (e.g active v placebo) and their responses to this compared.

Although these design features are intended to minimise bias and maximise predictability, they all challenge the fundamental principles of ethical research. The use of a control or placebo group means that some participants may receive a non-active intervention, which may significantly damage their well-being. For instance, an RCT looking at the effects of folic acid on neural tube development might involve the random allocation of women to either the folic acid intervention or the placebo. This might conceivably mean that the chances of neural tube disorders would be significantly higher in the non-intervention group. While the research design might be laudable, it arguably undermines the principles of beneficence, non-maleficence, fidelity, and justice. Moreover, if the double-blind requirement is also fulfilled, then veracity is undermined. Even if a new treatment is compared with an existing treatment, if there is a suspicion that one intervention is superior to another, then ethical doubts must creep in. Random allocation to treatment procedures is a cornerstone of RCTs and yet it challenges the right of self-determination. Consequently it carries ethical implications, since in true randomisation participants can express no preference about which intervention they receive, and they do not know what it is they are receiving. While the participants should have been fully aware of the possibility of being entered into any arm of the trial, allocation to the non-standard intervention may raise many unforeseen problems for the participants.

Matching participants on key criteria is not only methodologically difficult, but is arguably unjust. Variables that might influence the study's outcomes are identified and if they cannot be excluded, then participants are matched accordingly. This results in homogeneous groups, with potential participants being eliminated if they do not meet the inclusion criteria. This means that some potential participants are deprived of the potential benefits of entering the study. Moreover, RCT studies often use the best resources that do not reflect normal protocols. For example, Black (1996) recounts an RCT study of glue ear, in which operations were performed by highly experienced surgeons, when the standard hospital practice was to use junior surgeons.

Identical treatment of participants is also essential for the effective conduct of RCTs, yet it is virtually impossible to deliver the same care in the same way. Consider, for example, the 'changing child-birth' RCTs (e.g. Shields et al 1998). How can the researchers be sure that every participant in each of the treatment arms (traditional v midwifery-led care) received exactly the same level, type and nature of care? Each woman has different needs and it would be profession-ally as well as ethically irresponsible to be unreceptive to these, and simply to provide an unvarying package of treatment, irrespective of the evident needs of the women.

Such kudos is attached to RCTs and their results that the stakes are inevitably high. Where gains are to be made, there is always the potential for corruption, and indeed Coulter (1991) in an audit of trials carried out between 1977 and 1970, found serious flaws in 11%. Furthermore, he noted that some researchers deliberately distorted data for the purposes of academic and professional promotion and contaminated the study's design and conduct through inexperience and incompetence. Although these problems are not confined to RCTs, this nevertheless illustrates the way in which ethical proced-ures can be waived where vested interests are involved.

HOW WILL THE FINDINGS BE DISSEMINATED?

If research is to inform and improve midwifery practice, then it must be properly and widely disseminated in order that other practitioners can evaluate the findings and incorporate them appropriately into their own service delivery. There is a moral obligation on both the researchers to report and the practitioners to evaluate. Researchers are obliged to report because participants volunteer on the basis of the potential benefits that the research can achieve. Practitioners are obliged to evaluate because they are required to undertake best practice wherever possible. However, this can only be achieved if the research is fairly and properly recorded.

The current pressure on researchers in all areas to publish research means that there is a potential for bias and corruption. To comply with central government pressure for an increase in research output, it is conceivable that three types of problem might emerge:

1. Researchers might report incomplete research before the findings have been thoroughly verified.
2. Researchers might break up the data set up in order to increase the number of papers and in so doing might present a set of results that are distorted, clinically meaningless or not representative of the whole picture.
3. Researchers might fabricate data or 'massage' results.

Therefore, researchers have a responsibility to ensure that what is published is a full and fair account of the outcome of their research. The results should be interpreted as objectively as possible and the conclusions should not be extravagant. These points become difficult if a project has been sponsored by a government department or commercial organisation that has an investment in the outcome. In such cases it has been known for contradictory or unacceptable findings to be suppressed in order to protect the agency.

It is therefore important that the researcher retains the right to report accurately the results of sponsored work as long as the findings do not *unnecessarily* compromise the sponsor. As with all other aspects of research, confidentiality should not be breached in the report, and the identity of all participants should be protected unless they have given their written consent to the contrary.

As with all written work, plagiarism is absolutely unacceptable. If quotations or excerpts are to be used, appropriate authorisation and proper protocol should be observed. And, of course, the researcher should always be prepared to allow access to the raw data. Cravenness in this regard breeds suspicion, not only about the researcher's integrity, but also about both method and findings.

CONCLUSIONS

Any research using human subjects carries obligations to protect their rights, dignity and welfare. Midwifery, with its involvement with vulnerable client groups has a particular responsibility to follow appropriate ethical guidelines in order to safeguard the participants. This chapter has outlined where the major ethical obstacles arise in midwifery research. It must be emphasised that there are no definitive rules regarding ethical issues and their resolution; each problem requires negotiation, careful consideration and compromise. As a consequence the following points must be regarded as basic guidelines for conducting ethically acceptable research:

- Always observe the six principles of ethical research.
- Always obtain full and informed consent from participants.
- Always keep the dignity and welfare of the subjects paramount; never diminish, embarrass or compromise them.
- Always protect the participants' confidentiality and privacy.
- Ensure that the participants know that they can withdraw from the research at any time without sanction or compromising their care.
- Always consult with relevant authorities and committees to obtain the necessary approval before embarking on research. (Failure to do so might mean that the research cannot be published, which effectively renders it useless.)
- Always discuss with experienced independent others any methodological issues that might compromise the participants.
- Be as fair, accurate and objective as possible.

Openness, honesty and integrity breed trust and respect between professionals and client groups. Any profession wishing to pursue research must recognise that the privilege of research is earned through scrupulous behaviour and carries with it both ethical and moral obligations.

References

American Psychological Association 2002 Code of ethics. Online. Available: http://www.apa.org/ethics/code 2002.html

Black N 1996 Why we need observational studies to evaluate the effectiveness of health care. British Medical Journal 312:1215–1218

Brawley O W 1999 The study of untreated syphilis in the Negro male. International Journal of Radiation Oncology, Biology, Physics 40:5–8

British Psychological Society 2000 Code of ethics. Online. Available: http://bps.org.uk/about/rules5.cfm

Brown S J, Alexander J, Thomas P 1999 Feeding outcome in breast-fed term babies, supplemented by cup or bottle. Midwifery 15:92–96

Coolican H 1992 Research methods and statistics in psychology. Hodder & Stoughton, London

Corbie-Smith G et al 1999 Attitudes and beliefs of African Americans towards participation in medical research. Journal of General Internal Medicine 14:537–546

Coulter H L 1991 The controlled clinical trial: an analysis. Centre for Empirical Medicine, Washington DC

Department of Health 1993 Report of the Task Force on the Strategy for Research in Nursing Midwifery and Health Visiting. Department of Health, Leeds

Data Protection Act 1998 HMSO, London. Online. Available: http://www.hmso.gov.uk/acts/acts1998/19980029.htm

Eckstein S 2003 Manual for research committees, 6th edn. Cambridge University Press, Cambridge

Foy R, Parry J, McAvoy B 1998 Clinical trials in primary care. British Medical Journal 317:1168–1169

Gamble V N 1997 The Tuskegee Syphilis Study and women's health. Journal of the American Medical Women's Association 52:195–196

Harries U, Edwards J 1994 Gift or gain. Health Service Journal 104:26–27

Hicks C M 1992 Research in midwifery: are midwives their own worst enemies? Midwifery 8:12–18

Hicks C, Spurgeon P, Barwell F 2003 Changing childbirth: a pilot project. Journal of Advanced Nursing 42(6):617–628

Hofling C K et al 1966 An experimental study in nurse–physician relationships. Journal of Nervous and Mental Disease 143:171–180

International Confederation of Midwives 1993 International code of ethics for midwives. International Confederation of Midwives, London

International Council of Nurses 1996 Ethical guidelines for nursing research. ICN, Geneva

Ireland J et al 2000 Cord care practice in Scotland. Midwifery 16:237–245

Lydon-Rochelle M, Albers L 1993 Research trends in the Journal of Nurse-Midwifery 1987–1992. Journal of Nurse-Midwifery 38:343–348.

McCourt C, Pearce A 2000 Does continuity of carer matter to women from ethnic minority groups? Midwifery 16:145–154

McHaffie H 1998 Commentary—Gaining ethical approval: a necessity or an optional extra? Midwifery 14:101–104

Melender H-L, Lauri S 1999 Fears associated with pregnancy and childbirth—experiences of women who have recently given birth. Midwifery 15:177–182

Milgram S 1963 Behavioural study of obedience. Journal of Abnormal and Social Psychology 67:371–378

Milgram S 1974 Obedience to authority: an experimental view. Harper & Row, New York

Morin K et al 2002 Managing conflicts of interest in the conduct of clinical trials. Journal of the American Medical Association 287:78–84

Mosley C, Whittle C, Hicks C 2001 Method of supplementary feeding of pre-term babies and its impact on subsequent establishment of breast-feeding: a small scale pilot study using a randomised controlled trial. Midwifery 17:150–157

New B, Le Grand J 1996 Rationing in the NHS: principles and pragmatism. King's Fund, London

North Staffordshire Changing Childbirth Research Team 2000 A randomised study of midwifery caseload care and traditional 'shared care'. Midwifery 16:251–340

Office of the Inspector General 2000 Recruiting human subjects: pressures in industry-sponsored clinical research. Office of the Inspector General, Department of Health and Human Services, Washington DC

Parahoo K 1997 Nursing research: principles, process and issues. Macmillan, Basingstoke

Peckham M 1991 Research for health: a research and development strategy for the NHS. HMSO, London

Polgar S, Thomas S A 1992 Introduction to research in the health sciences. Churchill Livingstone, Melbourne

Polit D, Hungler B 1995 Nursing research: principles and methods, 5th edn. JB Lippincott, Pennsylvania

Renfrew M 2000 Developing high quality research in midwifery: lessons learned from the midwifery research data base MIRIAD. Midwifery 16:229–236

Robson C 1993 Real world research. Blackwell, Oxford

Sheehan A 1999 A comparison of two methods of breast-feeding education. Midwifery 15:274–282

Shields N et al 1998 Satisfaction with midwife-managed care in different time periods: a randomised controlled trial of 1299 women. Midwifery 14:85–93

Sibbald B, Roland M 1998 Why are randomised controlled trials important? British Medical Journal 316:201

Sjostrom H, Nilsson R 1972 Thalidomide and the power of the drug companies. Penguin, Harmondsworth

Spurgeon P, Hicks C, Barwell F 2001 Ante-natal, delivery and postnatal comparisons of maternal satisfaction with two pilot Changing Childbirth schemes, compared with a traditional model of care. Midwifery 17:123–132

Waldenstrom U, Nilsson C A 1997 A randomised controlled study of birth centre care versus standard maternity care: effects on women's health. Birth 24:17–26

Waldenstrom U, Turnbull D 1998 A systematic review comparing continuity of midwifery care with standard maternity services. British Journal of Obstetrics and Gynaecology 105:1160–1170

Whelan A, Lupton P 1998 Promoting successful breastfeeding among women with a low income. Midwifery 14:94–100

Wilkund H et al 2000 Somalis giving birth in Sweden: a challenge to culture and gender specific values and behaviours. Midwifery 16:105–115

Wilton T 1999 Towards a better understanding of the cultural roots of homophobia in order to provide a better midwifery service for lesbian clients. Midwifery 15:154–164

World Health Organisation 2000 Declaration of Helsinki. World Medical Association

Chapter **15**

Researching sensitive issues: a personal view

Hazel McHaffie

INTRODUCTION

Throughout their training, midwives are taught to identify a problem and attempt to solve it. Researchers, on the other hand, are encouraged to stand back, observe and note what is taking place but not to 'interfere' lest they influence the dynamics of any situation and jeopardise the integrity of their study. But researchers as well as clinicians are sometimes privy to confidences and information that may have a profound effect on them, and serious consequences for other people.

For researchers investigating areas where potentially damaging information is divulged, real dilemmas may arise. How far should they go in preserving confidences? When do their duties as healthcare practitioners supersede their obligations as researchers? At what point does danger to life or well-being take precedence over quality of the data produced? How far should they allow their own values, beliefs and interests to be compromised?

To some extent almost all research with human beings involves asking oneself just where the balance lies. Questions concern harm and benefit; privacy and confidentiality; informed consent and deception; and social control (Kelman 1982). There are social and moral obligations that relate both to the personal relationships a researcher develops with people in the field, and to the purpose and conduct of the study; for example, how much does a researcher disclose of his or her own agenda and experience? Does sharing personal detail bias respondents or facilitate an honest exchange? Encouraging respondents to gain insight into their feelings, or to re-live painful experiences may provide rich data but what happens to the respondent after the interview? How far does the interviewer's responsibility stretch in the therapeutic direction, especially if he or she has had no relevant training?

In studies on sensitive topics, the questions can become deeply searching. The usual basic and underlying issues are highlighted with particular clarity when seen against the backcloth of threat or secrecy. From the participants' point of view, there may be a risk of powerful emotions being generated or exposed, of loss of respect, and of shame, guilt or public exposure. For the researcher, taboos and restrictions may limit openness. As a consequence, researchers may sanitise their reports. Funding agencies may issue embargoes to suppress sensitive or potentially threatening findings. Gatekeepers may require the investigators to hide or disguise facts to accommodate the host institution's own agenda. Straightforward courtesy and sensitivity may dictate that a veil be drawn over parts of the research simply to protect the finer feelings of other human beings. If a subject is also topical, there is the additional risk of discomforting distortion by the media. Accordingly, much may be left unsaid.

Indeed, much *has* been left unsaid in the course of research carried out in sensitive areas over the years. Furthermore, serious academic attempts to 'tell it like it really is' have on occasions been thwarted because of the 'concealed micropolitics of research' (Punch 1986). Colleagues, editors and publishers have fought shy of contentious material. As a result, student researchers and others have not always benefited as they might from the wisdom gained from actual experience. This chapter attempts to address some of the issues raised by research of this nature.

SENSITIVE TOPICS AND THE DEGREE OF THREAT

Sensitive areas for research include both topics that touch deep-seated emotions and those that involve behaviours that are intimate, incriminating or possibly discreditable. Although all research may have some costs to those participating, in sensitive areas the price is recognised as particularly high and likely to occur. A substantial degree of threat exists for those being studied and there is a corresponding burden to be carried by the investigator.

Such research may raise methodological problems as well as ethical or legal ones, and the difficulties may occur at almost any stage of the research process. That is not to say that such research should not be undertaken, although some researchers have suggested that certain areas should not be subjected to close scrutiny.

The study of taboos by anthropologists and of privacy by sociologists show how important it is for a culture that certain areas of personal and social life should be specially protected. Intimacy cannot exist where everything is disclosed, sanctuary cannot be sought where no place is inviolate, integrity cannot be seen to be maintained—and therefore cannot in certain cases be maintained—without protection from illegitimate pressures. (MacIntyre 1982)

However, a cogent argument can be made for research into people's private lives. It can be justified not only on the basis that it will substantially increase knowledge, but also on the grounds that the process itself may be of benefit to the respondents themselves. In my own work among mothers with very low birth weight babies, the women frequently commented on the therapeutic effect of sharing their anxieties, anger and frustration. Some volunteered that talking through these issues with me helped them to keep tensions with their partners in check and to avoid actually harming the baby. Sometimes catharsis is more desirable than sanctuary (Lee & Renzetti 1993). The skill lies in achieving a healthy balance between maximum validity and benefit, and minimum harm.

In conventional positivist theory '[t]he investigator's task is to discover that which is hidden or kept secret by subjects (or that which remains unknown to them) and to hold these discovered truths, these facts, to the light of scientific scrutiny. Secrecy has no permanent place in this form of scientific enterprise' (Mitchell 1991). But a moment's sober reflection will reveal that secrecy pervades human relations and it would be arrogant to believe that a researcher either could or should uncover all that a respondent has chosen to conceal from others. The degree of disclosure remains a matter of continual negotiation and is to some extent dependent on the nature of the relationship established; the identity, perceived role and skill of the researcher; and the sense of control, self-esteem and comfort of the respondent.

The perception of harm among the respondents themselves may well be different from that of their gatekeepers, or society in general. To incur the displeasure or sanction of any of these groups is to jeopardise the value of the research findings. The experiences, values, perceptions and agendas of people will vary and the onus is on the researcher to gain insight into the sensitivities of others and to minimise the onslaught to such feelings.

To some extent the degree of threat is a matter of personal assessment: what is threatening to one person may be innocuous to another. What a gatekeeper considers sensitive material may not be perceived as such by the person investigating the topic. The challenge is to anticipate how others may perceive an investigation, and to build in benefits for those who are willing to participate.

There are, however, commonly accepted social contexts that may lead one to anticipate that certain topics may be especially sensitive. Research in the fields of child abuse, sexual 'deviance' or illegal drug selling is likely to be fraught with problems of threat and fear of recrimination. Yet even sometimes seemingly innocuous enquiries can unearth strong threats because of the idiosyncratic experiences of some of the participants that the researcher could not have anticipated; for example, a study of first-time mothers may lead to a respondent disclosing experience of previous abortion or of a surrogacy arrangement that for her carry a risk of unwelcome discovery. For this individual the subject is sensitive, but in ways that the researcher could not have anticipated.

It sometimes happens that even when sensitivities have been respected, the perceived harm exceeds expectations, for example, a respondent may divulge highly sensitive information during the course of an interview with a skilled researcher but subsequently regret the 'moment of weakness', and feel hostile towards the person who achieved the disclosure. Where there is a continuing relationship between the two, this can be uncomfortable and inhibiting for both parties. If there is no further contact the respondent can be left with unresolved tensions that may be damaging to self-esteem, confidence or comfort.

PREPARATION OF THE RESEARCHER

My own experiences as a researcher have exposed me to a number of situations that have involved much heart searching. I am persuaded that there are few definitive answers—each situation needs to be assessed carefully and minutely. But I believe that researchers are more credible, and perceived as more trustworthy, if they honestly declare the cause of their anxiety and the action taken, rather than covering up the problem that has arisen. Textbooks on research methods rarely address the reality of such dilemmas. Indeed, as Punch (1986) has commented, such research:

involves an inexhaustible variety of settings and an endless range of situational exigencies for which ready-made recipes do not exist. The conduct of the researcher, and the outcomes of research, are vulnerable to unique developments in the field and to dramatic predicaments that can often be solved only situationally.

But sweeping the issues under the carpet is not the way to future enlightenment. Every researcher should at least be alive to the issues and prepared in some measure for the decisions and their justification. In the very first piece of research I carried out, I was challenged fairly early into its design to consider what I would do if exactly such situations arose. The investigation involved my going out and talking to mothers of very low birth weight babies. The interviews spanned the period of hospitalisation and the 3 months after the baby's discharge from a neonatal unit. They took place for the most part in the mothers' own homes. My challenger was a psychiatrist on an ethics committee who saw this novice researcher, out in the community, seeing and hearing worrying things, party to burdensome information, and totally unprepared for dealing with it. I was asked, kindly and wisely, to outline my line of communication in such circumstances. On many occasions during the conduct of that study, I had cause to be grateful that I had been forced to address these possibilities from the outset. I have remained indebted to that psychiatrist for his insight and commitment to ensuring that research was not detrimental to the well-being of its subjects or to me, even though the study was exploratory and involved no interventions.

There is a common misperception that only research involving things like radioactive isotopes or experimental interventions really requires REC approval. This is not so. Even in a study as apparently benign as mine there was a form of intervention: my presence and my questioning. It had consequences, not as evidently potentially harmful as powerful drugs, maybe, but consequences nonetheless.

Because researchers fear that some areas are too sensitive to study openly, research has occasionally been carried out in a covert way. Probably the most well known example is Humphrey's (1970) *Tearoom Trade* study of impersonal sex in public places. Humphrey conducted fieldwork among men having impersonal sex in public facilities, and acted as a 'watch queen'. This enabled him to offer his services as a lookout for intruders, in exchange for the opportunity to observe sexual activity. By means of recording licence numbers of the men's cars, he traced their names and addresses and then, with changed hairstyle and form of dress, visited them at home as part of a 'social health survey'. The richness of data obtained from his work may be beyond doubt, but many people, myself included, have serious misgivings about the ethics of such deceit (Beauchamp et al 1982).

Most midwifery research appears innocuous by comparison, but the same rights and ethical principles need to be considered. In field-work with certain topics, there seems no way around the predica-ment that truly informed consent may 'kill many a project stone dead' (Punch 1986), or be unworkable in the given circumstances. Nevertheless the benefits of knowledge must be carefully weighed against the consequences to the respondents and those closely asso-ciated with them.

However, the fact that certain research studies pose complex ethical problems does not mean that they should not be attempted. As Sieber & Stanley (1988) have argued, some of society's most pressing social questions are those commonly thought to be 'sensitive'. Ignoring them is not a responsible approach to science. Shying away from them simply because they are controversial is also an avoidance of respon-sibility. But if researchers do embark on such studies, it is imperative that they do not ignore the methodological difficulties inherent in such work (Lee & Renzetti 1993).

THE COSTS

It is not just to the respondents that harm may accrue. There are con-siderable costs to be borne by investigators and it must be remem-bered that 'empirical studies serve not only to create knowledge. They are also the hard currency with which researchers negotiate their careers, and often play an important role in the construction of personal identity and self-esteem' (Frost & Stablein 1992a).

Researchers themselves may be put at risk because of the nature of their enquiry. Punch (1986) catalogued studies where researchers had been subjected to verbal and physical violence, public caricature, legal challenge, or eviction from the field. There were instances of fieldworkers going insane, panicking or getting cold feet and never embarking on the fieldwork, of 'obstructionist gatekeepers, vacillat-ing sponsors, factionalism in the field setting forcing the researcher to choose sides, organisational resistance, respondents subverting the research role, sexual shenanigans, and disputes about publication and veracity of findings' (Punch 1986).

Glazer (1972) analysed the dynamics of many researchers' encounters with respondents, exploring the balance of reciprocity, trust, tolerance, friendship, and identification. He found that researchers were confronted by social injustice, hostility, condemnation, a sense of guilt and other powerful reactions. Compared with studies set in dangerous and shadowy social contexts, midwifery research can appear relatively tame and free from problems, but the same issues and conflicts are pertinent nonetheless.

I have had good reason to fear for my personal safety as a result of entering, alone and unprotected, homes where violence was the norm. Working in the area of HIV infection, I took on board some of the stigma and rejection levelled against those infected with the virus. Psychological damage can be as draining as the fear of physical harm. Painful and alarming disclosures can be extremely wearing. Being told about illegal or immoral actions; seeing behaviours that jeopardise the safety of vulnerable people; being sworn to secrecy about some highly damaging information; all leave the researcher burdened. Personal integrity may be compromised. The strength of one's commitment to scholarly enquiry may be seriously questioned.

I have lost count of the number of times a respondent has said, 'I haven't told another living soul about that'. It can be enormously therapeutic for someone to unburden themselves to a person who says the information disclosed will go no further, but the consequences for the researcher can be onerous. Difficult decisions have to be made. Where do responsibilities begin and end?

INDIVIDUAL RESPONSIBILITY

Since there are often no right answers, it would be unhelpful merely to catalogue points for consideration or to outline a framework for behaviours. Rote learning will only take an individual so far. The unexpected, the perplexing and the threatening situation will still potentially present problems. In order to deal with these well, the researcher needs an understanding of the underlying issues. It is beyond the scope of this chapter to address every ethical, legal, professional and practical problem that may arise when conducting research into sensitive issues. Instead, a series of short journeys into real-life fieldwork with a sensitive component will be undertaken. No attempt will be made to analyse each situation comprehensively;

rather the illustrations will provide a starting point in the process of considering the arguments and viewpoints. It is important to remember that each individual researcher must be able to give an adequate account of his or her behaviour and defend chosen decisions and actions. It is part of being professionally accountable.

Example 1

Irene was 22 years old, living with her boyfriend, Tom, in a very run down part of a large city. Tom, an unemployed labourer, was the second of three sons. Both his brothers were in prison for crimes of violence—murder and mugging respectively. Irene's own mother refused to visit them at home since she considered the neighbourhood both dangerous and beneath her, but Tom's family dropped in frequently.

Irene's pregnancy was not planned but until 28 weeks it was clinically uneventful, then raised blood pressure necessitated Irene's admission to hospital. An emergency caesarean section was carried out 2 weeks later when her pre-eclampsia could not be controlled. The baby girl, Cheryl, weighed 1277 grams and was in good condition at birth, requiring only headbox oxygen. But Irene found the whole experience of having an operation terrifying and was convinced she herself would die.

Her first view of Cheryl was through a haze of drugs and she pronounced her 'quite nice', but once the medication was withdrawn, she was horrified by the child's appearance: in Irene's opinion Cheryl resembled a 'half dead bird' and she was revolted and extremely loath to touch her. Gradually, over the 8 weeks that Cheryl remained in the neonatal unit, Irene found she quite enjoyed holding the baby, provided she was well wrapped up in blankets and fast asleep, but awake and crying she terrified her mother. Tom, however, well used to dealing with a stream of small nephews and nieces, appeared quite at home in the neonatal unit and handled the baby with pleasure and confidence. This irritated Irene. Her relationship with Tom had always been tempestuous and there were now frequent arguments, resulting, on several occasions in one or other of them storming out of the nursery in anger.

Irene saw little of her mother and declared that she had no one to confide in except me. Indeed, she welcomed the opportunity to be involved in a project that gave her ongoing opportunities to talk to someone she perceived to be non-authoritarian. Over the months of her participation in the study, she continued to be preoccupied with the child's 'ugliness', believing there was something very abnormal about her. Medically Cheryl's condition was uncomplicated—her only problem was a poor toleration of feeds. In real terms to Irene her problems were manifested in excessive vomiting at feed times, the baby going blue in the face and fighting for breath. Perversely, she felt, Cheryl fed beautifully for everyone else.

Such was her terror, that throughout the whole 8 weeks, Irene never completed a feed with Cheryl, always passing her on to a neonatal nurse with a variety of excuses for why she could not remain in the nursery. But since she believed the nurses had certain expectations of mothers, she took care to use different excuses and apply to different members of staff for help. She considered it would have been quite unacceptable to tell the health care team that she was unwilling to feed her baby. As a researcher, I presented no such threat; she had been assured that I would respect confidences. I gave no advice, and had taken no part in saving the baby's life. As a result she was able to confide that she 'hated' the child and did not want her home.

On my first visit after Cheryl's discharge I found a highly anxious Irene. She and Tom did not go to bed at night but slept uneasily on the floor beside Cheryl's cot. Both were seriously perturbed by her 'screeching', which went on sometimes for as long as 5 hours. Neither was prepared to be left alone with the baby, fearful that they might harm her if there was no one else to keep them in check.

Against this background, I was more than a little concerned when Irene failed to answer my ring at her door 1 month after she had taken Cheryl home. The usual repeat visits, after leaving notes through the door, simply established that someone had been into the house between my calls, but there was no word of what had happened to make Irene break our appointment. She had repeatedly discussed with me her hatred towards the baby, and how near she had come to harming her seriously. If her word was true, no one except me knew about this. I felt profoundly troubled.

What was I to do? On the one hand, my contract as a researcher made me respect her confidences. I had given a solemn undertaking to do so. And the quality of my research was at stake: if I intervened I was substantially influencing the situation and any further data collected from her could be invalid. Moreover, how would my clinical colleagues react to 'interference' from outside? They were after all responsible for the health and well-being of this family and I was on their territory. But on the other hand, I was seriously alarmed about the welfare of this child. Was she lying dead in a gas oven? Had Irene also done harm to herself? My responsibility as a human being and as a caring nurse seemed to make it impossible to walk away and do nothing.

The advice of the REC proved enormously helpful. They had required me to specify my lines of communication in the event of a situation arising where I was seriously concerned for the welfare of the family. I was able simultaneously to respect the detail of Irene's confidences and to alert the health care team to a potential problem. The agreed course of action was that I phoned my academic supervisor who was a consultant neonatologist. He then rang Irene's GP and asked that the health visitor investigate Irene's absence. I was sufficiently concerned about Irene myself to continue to call, hoping to find her in. My persistence was eventually rewarded. Both mother and baby were alive. The endless screaming had antagonised an elderly neighbour, who had threatened to report the parents to the police for abusing the child. Irene fled to friends' homes. There she abdicated responsibility for bathing and feeding Cheryl, leaving it to her calmer friends. Her flight had helped her to cope, and the passage of time had improved her own ability to look after her larger, more coordinated baby.

Example 2

I first became acutely aware of the baggage a researcher brings to any encounter when I was working with people who had become infected with HIV. Because of its close association with death and sex, this is a particularly sensitive area in which to practise.

As part of my enquiry I interviewed key professionals throughout the UK. For one such session I was requested to go to an HIV clinic in a large hospital. Finding no signs to this clinic, I approached the staff in an ordinary outpatient clinic for advice. I was totally unprepared for their reaction. Not only did they not know, but they did not want to know. They referred me to another building. In all five encounters I had with staff in different departments in that hospital in the course of my search for the clinic, I felt the same sense of discomfort. I met with outright scorn, conspiratorial whispering, and public humiliation. My failure to state the purpose of my visit began as an accident, but became deliberate. Much as I smarted under the reactions, it gave me a salutary experience akin to that of a patient attending for testing for the first time. But unlike them, I was hundreds of miles from my home, extremely unlikely to meet anyone I knew, and not actually seeking a test. Nonetheless it was still a painful experience.

As part of preparation for this study I became much more aware of the use of language. In the world of HIV and AIDS, words and expressions in common usage may acquire totally different connotations. Common assumptions about gender, affiliations and attitudes may all be misplaced. At times my own value systems were competing with those of my respondents. It was impossible to become cognisant of all such differences and pitfalls in the space of a few weeks, but in recognising my own naivety I was better able to recognise the pitfalls, and avoid some of the mistakes. It was still difficult to deal with the accounts of blatant discrimination and injustice and insensitive management of individuals, but I was more aware of my own reactions and the effect I might have on respondents and on the data.

Indeed, to some extent, being brought face to face with my own attitudes and feelings helped me to understand what respondents talked about in disclosing their own problems in this area. I knew what interviewees, who were also health care professionals, meant when they talked about being offended by shock tactics, being discomposed by blatant references to unusual sexual practices, being ambivalent about accepting an invitation to a client's home, and feeling that they were being asked to condone everything. For those clinicians whose experience has been extensive and who have developed a special skill in this area, it can be difficult to identify with the new recruit for whom this seems like a disturbing and dangerous world, but their perspective is legitimate too, and in-depth discussions with specialists helped me to keep a balance and to understand their world.

This was the first research I had carried out in an area of practice with which I was not clinically familiar. There are problems as well as benefits to entering a sensitive field as a novice. Although I had read extensively on the subject and talked to specialists informally as well as on working parties, it was possible I would simply fail to understand what was being said. I might inadvertently offend or upset respondents because I was unaware of the nuances of this speciality. On the positive side, I was able to ask for explanations of the obvious and I could probe for understanding of the taken-for-granted things, which a more expert clinician could not do with any degree of credibility.

Because of all the potential problems, care needed to be taken to verify the study findings. An important part of the design of this enquiry involved testing the results with a variety of groups of people to be confident that an accurate and scientific analysis was achieved.

Opportunities were built in to enable practitioners, educators, managers, and clients to discuss the results and determine whether they represented reality as they perceived it. I repeatedly checked my interpretations against the yardstick of experience.

Example 3

Asking clinicians about their practices and beliefs in relation to withholding or withdrawing treatment from extremely sick neonates was guaranteed to be emotionally taxing. This is a difficult environment to enter. The tensions and stresses of staff working in intensive care units are well documented. I found myself caught more than once in emotional crossfire about which I could only dimly discern the causes. When I was intent on cultivating trust and building up rapport with the medical and nursing staff, I found it disconcerting to feel the tensions even when they actually stemmed from administrative problems or personality clashes. It was all too easy to take them personally. There was too a very real danger of overidentification with respondents, which I had to keep to the forefront of my mind.

Nor was the nature of the subject an easy one to explore. There were many sensitivities wrapped up in its boundaries. A number of clinicians have already experienced the trauma of being taken to court by parents who hold a grievance against them for the death or impaired life of their child. Legal backing appears uncertain. Furthermore, media programmes designed to bring these matters to public attention do little to reassure clinicians. There are threats inherent in asking them to share their experiences on such delicate matters.

Methodologically, much careful thought was needed in the design of this project. I considered it was important to spend time establishing trust in each unit before interviewing staff. Part of this preparation involved my being present at all hours of the day and night, at weekends, as well as over public holidays. Words were chosen carefully and the term 'euthanasia' was avoided. Respondents were encouraged to detail their own experiences of specific cases to give them a sense of control and confidence in their own coherence. Access to staff and the selection of representative respondents was carried out in careful conjunction with the practitioners and in line with clinical commitments and demands. But for me, there was a price to be paid. I was a visitor in close knit teams: an outsider. I had to be vigilant not to overstep the bounds of my welcome. The dividing line between involvement and intrusion required repeated testing.

And there was a heavy weight to be carried emotionally in conducting an enquiry which involved interviewing many professionals. It was burdensome to be in receipt of frequent stories involving powerful emotions. These included not only those involving neonates, but also accounts of the deaths of close relatives, the burdens of impairment and the stress of life events of various kinds. Some of these touched raw nerves of my own that I had thought were healed. An important feature of in-depth interviewing is that the researcher needs to concentrate totally throughout the discussion, weaving in past information and taking account of additional and serendipitous keys to the respondent's feelings and view. But this requires clarity of thinking and a freedom from distraction. It is vital to come to each encounter with a freshness and keen interest in what this new individual will contribute to understanding of this topic.

I quickly learned that being up half the night, and working long stretches without a break, dulled my senses. I had to limit the number of interviews I conducted concurrently. I had to forget pride in my own ability to survive a gruelling schedule and learn to be kinder to myself. Only then could I give what was needed to each research encounter. In previous studies where profound emotions had been exposed, I had nominated colleagues to listen to what burdened me and thereby rid myself of tensions that could inhibit effective future interviewing. With this enquiry the information received was of a greater sensitivity. I had given careful assurances to all those involved that I would do all in my power to safeguard the identity of each institution as well as each individual. A sense of absolute safety was vital to the success of the enquiry. I had to learn to deal with the psychological burden using inner resources and relaxing outside pursuits. However, much of the time spent data collecting, I was away from home and my usual sources of refreshment. New techniques had to be developed; other outlets for tension found.

SOME FUNDAMENTALS

These few examples are merely illustrative of the reality of researching in the sensitive areas. As Glazer (1972) expressed it:

> The satisfaction, excitement, frustrations, challenges, and agonies of field research are not time bound. They are as real and relevant today as when they occurred … The questions continue to be fundamental … crucial and must be constantly expressed, discusssed and evaluated. Those who would participate in the adventures of

research must continually confront the most challenging questions of scientific ethics and social responsibility. For we are deeply 'involved in mankind'.

Health care professionals are the envy of many other researchers. An enormously rich field for enquiry is open to them, and they are, indeed 'deeply involved in mankind'. Where they understand intimately the nuances of the situations they are investigating, they can bring special skills and an extra dimension to both collection and analysis. On occasions there may be a conflict between the demands of academia and professional instinct. But a primary loyalty towards the greater good of the population served by the health care service should be sufficient motivation to compel them to examine the research endeavour, and move towards more openness and honesty.

Although definitive answers to any dilemma are elusive, there are certain fundamental prerequisites relating to respect for respondents and responsible stewardship of data, as the previous chapter has outlined (see also Beauchamp et al 1982, Boruch & Cecil 1983, Frost & Stablein 1992b, Hunt 1989, Lee & Renzetti 1993, Punch 1986, Sieber 1993). Careful thought must be given to the design and conduct of the enquiry, to the fieldwork experience, to the analysis of the data, and to the dissemination of findings. At all levels, sensitivities may be offended and quality jeopardised. Awareness of the issues and rehearsal of the options may go some way towards minimising any harm.

I share Punch's (1986) view that 'openness, debate, individual responsibility, and professional accountability on the conduct of research are more likely to spell out a sensible and healthy approach to the moral dilemmas in fieldwork than regulation'. Codes tend to be too vague and may indeed create unnecessary barriers. Rigid standards and sanctions cannot be imposed in a world where there are no clearly definable ways of calculating costs and benefits. Research ethics are not clear-cut matters that conform to such laws or guidelines, but open debate of the issues can both take account of fundamental principles and allow for the vagaries of specific situations. Coming clean about the realities of fieldwork experience may well go some way towards achieving a greater integrity.

ACKNOWLEDGEMENTS

I am indebted to Kenneth Boyd and Jennifer Sleep for their helpful comments on the first draft of this chapter.

References

Beauchamp T L et al (eds) 1982 Ethical issues in social science research. Johns Hopkins University Press, Baltimore

Boruch R F, Cecil J S 1983 Solutions to ethical and legal problems in social research. Academic Press, New York

Frost P J, Stablein R E 1992a Lessons from the journeys. In: Frost P J, Stablein R E (eds) Doing exemplary research. Sage, London, p 270–292

Frost P J, Stablein R E 1992b Doing exemplary research. Sage, London

Glazer M 1972 The research adventure: promise and problems of field work. Random House, London

Humphrey L 1970 Tearoom trade: impersonal sex in public places. Aldine, London

Hunt J C 1989 Psychoanalytic aspects of fieldwork. Sage, London

Kelman H C 1982 Ethical issues in different social science methods. In: Beauchamp T L et al (eds) 1982 Ethical issues in social science research. Johns Hopkins University Press, Baltimore, p 40–48

Lee R M, Renzetti C M 1993 The problems of researching sensitive topics: an overview and introduction. In: Lee R M, Renzetti C M (eds) Researching sensitive topics. Sage, London, p 3–13

MacIntyre A 1982 Risk, harm, and benefit assessment as instruments of moral evaluation. In: Beauchamp T L et al (eds) 1982 Ethical issues in social science research. Johns Hopkins University Press, Baltimore, p 175–189

Mitchell R G Jr 1991 Secrecy and disclosure in fieldwork. In: Shaffir W B, Stebbins R A (eds) Experiencing fieldwork: an insider view of qualitative research. Sage, London, p 97–108

Punch M 1986 The politics and ethics of fieldwork. Sage, London

Sieber J E 1993 The ethics and politics of sensitive research. In: Lee R M, Renzetti C M (eds) Researching sensitive topics. Sage, London, p 14–26

Sieber J E, Stanley B 1988 Ethical and professional dimensions of socially sensitive research. American Psychology 43:49–55

Index

ELSEVIER

B*f***M Books** *for* **Midwives**

**CHURCHILL
LIVINGSTONE**

Mosby

**THE PRACTISING
MIDWIFE**

🌸 **Baillière Tindall**

MIDWIFERY PUBLISHERS OF CHOICE FOR GENERATIONS

For many years and through several identities we have catered for
professional needs in midwifery education and practice. Leading publishers
of major textbooks such as *Myles Textbook for Midwives* and *Mayes' Midwifery:
a Textbook for Midwives*, our expertise spreads across both books and journals
to offer a comprehensive resource for midwives at all stages of their careers.

Find out how we can provide you with the right book at the right time by
exploring our website, **www.elsevierhealth.com/midwifery** or requesting
a midwifery catalogue from Health Professions Marketing, Elsevier, 32
Jamestown Road, Camden, London, NW1 7BY, UK Tel: 020 7424 4200;
Fax: 020 7424 4420.

We are always keen to expand our midwifery list so if you have an idea for
a new book please contact Mary Seager, Senior Commissioning Editor at
Elsevier, The Boulevard, Langford Lane, Kidlington, Oxford, OX5 1GB, UK
(m.seager@elsevier.com).

Have you joined yet?
Sign up for e-Alert to get the latest news and information.

Register for eAlert at www.elsevierhealth.com/eAlert Information direct to your Inbox

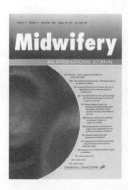

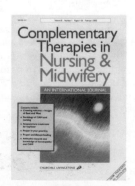